Phoebe

With this in view, small print has been used for matter which may definitely be included in the last category. In attempting to combine these three factors, a somewhat larger book than is usual for nurses has resulted. However, this has not been used as an excuse to produce an expensive work, and every effort has been made to keep its cost as low as possible.

I must express my gratitude to the late Mr. J. Rawlings Elliot, F.P.S., D.B.A., Chief Pharmacist to St. Bartholomew's Hospital, for the very great assistance he has been to me, not only in checking all the pharmaceutical details but also for many valuable suggestions. Without his help, the work could not have been completed.

My thanks are also due to Mr. T. Clare of Edward Arnold Ltd. for his courtesy and help in its production.

LONDON, 1943
W. GORDON SEARS

## PREFACE TO THE FIFTH EDITION

WITHOUT altering the general form of the book an endeavour has been made to bring this work up to date by including as many of the better known new drugs as possible and excluding some of the older ones which are rarely used.

In most instances the metric doses have been included and proprietary names have been placed in inverted commas in order to give some guidance in the present maze of inconsistent terminology. To attempt to include all the drugs which a nurse may encounter would be impossible. In cases of doubt she should remember that the British National Formulary and The Extra Pharmacopoeia (Martindale) are excellent works of reference.

I would, once again, like to thank Miss M. M. Rogers, F.P.S., Chief Pharmacist to Mile End Hospital for her valuable advice and for her help in reading the proofs.

LONDON, 1962
W. GORDON SEARS

# PREFACE TO THE FIRST EDITION

In *Medicine for Nurses* I included a short section on Materia Medica which was not intended to be more than a summary containing some essential facts likely to be asked in an examination.

I have, however, felt that nurses required something more comprehensive which would fulfil two purposes. The first, a book which would link up drugs and therapeutics with physiology, and which would be reasonably readable. The second, a work containing sufficient information to be useful for reference after examinations have been completed.

Nurses are constantly handling drugs to which they can find no reference in their ordinary text-books, and a spirit of enquiry is so often manifest, as Tutors and Ward Sisters will know, that I have not hesitated to include as many drugs as possible in the space at my disposal.

Materia Medica in its old-fashioned sense which deals with the various vegetable preparations and their botanical origin is of little importance to the nurse. On the other hand, the modern confusion of proprietary preparations, with and without official names, is a most difficult subject to comprehend, but at the same time is extremely important. Many of the more familiar proprietary preparations have, therefore, been mentioned.

Some stress has been laid on therapeutic procedures, signs of over-dosage and points which the nurse can observe or has to carry out for herself.

I would emphasize that this work, like my others, is not intended to be just put into a nurse's hands for her to learn the subject for an examination. The intention is that she should learn from it what it is necessary for her to know under the guidance of a competent teacher, for a nurse in training requires a teacher to indicate:

1. What she should learn for her examinations.
2. What she should read for her own interest.
3. What is included merely for reference.

© W. GORDON SEARS 1962

| First Published | . | . | . | . | . | 1943 |
| Reprinted | . | . | 1943, 1944 (twice), | | | 1945 |
| Second Edition | . | . | . | . | . | 1947 |
| Reprinted | . | . | . | . | . | 1948 |
| Third Edition | . | . | . | . | . | 1955 |
| Reprinted | . | . | . | . | . | 1958 |
| Fourth Edition | . | . | . | . | . | 1959 |
| Fifth Edition | . | . | . | . | . | 1962 |

*Printed in Great Britain by*
*Robert Cunningham and Sons Ltd., Alva*

# MATERIA MEDICA
# FOR NURSES

## A TEXT-BOOK OF
## DRUGS AND THERAPEUTICS

BY

### W. GORDON SEARS
M.D. (Lond.), M.R.C.P. (Lond.)
PHYSICIAN, MILE END HOSPITAL, LONDON
EXAMINER TO THE GENERAL NURSING COUNCIL FOR ENGLAND AND WALES

FIFTH EDITION

LONDON
EDWARD ARNOLD (PUBLISHERS) LTD

# MATERIA MEDICA FOR NURSES

# CONTENTS

# CHAPTER 1

# INTRODUCTION

The subject of Drugs and their uses is a very large one and has many branches. It is constantly expanding and, while new drugs are being discovered, others are falling into disuse.

## Definitions

1. The term *Materia Medica* may be used to include the whole subject.

2. A *Drug* is any substance taken into the body or applied to its surface for the prevention or treatment of disease.

3. *Pharmacy* is the art of preparing drugs in the various forms suitable for their administration, such as tinctures and extracts. Included in pharmacy is the practice of *Dispensing* which involves the compounding of preparations such as pills, mixtures and ointments from their various constituents.

4. *Pharmacology* deals with the mode of action of various drugs. It endeavours to explain on which organs of the body a drug acts and exactly how it operates. It is, therefore, closely united with physiology. For example, pharmacology explains how digitalis acts on the bundle of His in the heart, and slows the rate of the ventricle in auricular (atrial) fibrillation.
Drugs given in excessive amounts are liable to act as poisons, the study of which is called *Toxicology*.

5. *Therapeutics* is the art of using remedies in the treatment of disease. It embraces all the methods employed in the management and care of a patient whereby we endeavour to aid Nature in restoring the individual to health. Included also are the efforts made to relieve the patient's symptoms even if the disease cannot be cured, i.e. remedies may be (*a*) symptomatic or (*b*) curative.

### The British Pharmacopœia

The British Pharmacopœia (B.P.) is a list of "official" drugs and their doses published by the General Medical Council. It lays down the chemical standard which must be maintained in the manufacture of all drugs labelled "B.P." and is revised from time to time.

**The British Pharmaceutical Codex** (B.P.C.) is an "unofficial" work published by the Pharmaceutical Society of Great Britain which acts as a supplement to the B.P. and contains a number of other drugs and useful preparations.

**The British National Formulary** (B.N.F.) is a handbook which includes those drugs and preparations in common use, and is widely employed both in hospital and general practice as a basis for prescribing. There are also many useful notes on drugs which a nurse may well study.

Some hospitals have pharmacopœias prepared for their own convenience but they are all based on the B.P., B.P.C. or B.N.F.

**Proprietary Preparations.** In addition to the official and semi-official preparations, there are an enormous number of drugs prepared and sold by firms of manufacturing chemists all over the world. Some of them are very valuable, others are more or less useless, but it is only fair to say that many advances in therapeutics and the introduction of useful new drugs are due to the research and enterprise of these commercial undertakings. A number of these preparations ultimately become "official" and are included in the B.P., usually under a different name.

This is often very confusing because a drug is known for some years by its proprietary name and only later does the "official" term come into general use. For example, phenobarbitone became the "official" name for 'Luminal.'

(N.B.—They are denoted in the present text in inverted commas.)

### Terminology

One of the most difficult and confusing aspects of the subject to the beginner is the terminology used in the naming of drugs. In the first place it must be understood that therapeutic substances are of very varied origin.

**1. Vegetable.** Drugs may be obtained from various parts of many plants such as their leaves, roots, seeds, flowers, fruit or bark. Resins and some oils are also obtained from vegetable sources.

The modern tendency has been to extract the active principles from medicinal plants rather than to use the actual plants. There are, however, some well-known exceptions to this rule—e.g. (*a*) The use of senna pods to make the laxative, senna tea. (*b*) The use of powdered digitalis leaves (*Digitalis folia*) in the treatment of heart disease.

The two most important types of active principles extracted are:

(*a*) Alkaloids.

(*b*) Glycosides.

*Alkaloids.* These are usually highly active substances which are only used in very small doses. They contain nitrogen and their names generally terminate in -INE (in Latin -INA) thus:

> Morphine is an alkaloid of opium.
> Strychnine ,, ,, ,, nux vomica.
> Atropine ,, ,, ,, belladonna.
> Nicotine ,, ,, ,, tobacco.

*Glycosides* or *Glucosides.* These are very potent vegetable substances in the formation of which glucose, or some other sugar, takes part.

> Digoxin is a glycoside of digitalis.

The names of the glycosides terminate in -IN, although not every substance ending in this way is a glycoside, e.g. liquid paraffin is a mineral oil.

**2. Mineral.** This group includes well-known natural substances such as iron, bismuth, mercury and common chemical compounds like Epsom salts (magnesium sulphate), Glauber's salt (sodium sulphate) and various compounds of lime (calcium) and phosphorus (phosphates).

**3. Animal.** This term applies in particular to vaccines, sera, gland extracts, hormones and similar preparations.

**4. Synthetic.** The term "synthetic" is used to describe a large number of drugs, some of them very complicated in composition, which are prepared in chemical laboratories (e.g. the sulphonamides). The composition of many natural substances is also known, and some can be prepared chemically as well as being obtained from their natural sources. For example, adrenaline can be obtained from the suprarenal gland, but is more economically manufactured by ordinary chemical processes.

**5. Antibiotics.** These drugs play a very important part in the modern treatment of infections and consist of anti-bacterial substances derived from various moulds. They may be defined as chemical substances produced by micro-organisms, which prevent the growth of other micro-organisms. The best known examples are penicillin, strepto-mycin, the tetracyclines and chloramphenicol.

### Classification of drugs

It is convenient in a text-book to consider drugs acting on the various systems of the body together. It is also useful to classify them in general terms which indicate their main action. Although individual drugs will be dealt with in appropriate chapters the following definitions in common use may be found helpful.

Analgesics and anodyne drugs are used to relieve pain.

Antacids neutralize hydrochloric acid in the stomach.

Anthelmintics are used in the treatment of intestinal worms.

Anticoagulants such as heparin and 'Dindevan' diminish the clotting power of the blood.

Anticonvulsants are used in the treatment of epilepsy and other states in which irritation of the brain results in fits or convulsions; e.g. phenobarbitone.

Antidepressants stimulate the higher centres of the brain. They may cause wakefulness and a temporary feeling of well-being; e.g. amphetamine.

Antidiabetic drugs. In addition to insulin, the oral hypo-glycaemic agents tolbutamide and chlorpropamide ('Dia-binese') lower the blood sugar in diabetes.

Antihistamines counteract the action of histamine, a substance liberated in the tissues in a number of allergic conditions such as hay fever and urticaria.

Antipruritics are drugs which relieve itching.

Diuretics increase the secretion of urine.

Hæmopoietic drugs stimulate the formation of red cells e.g. vitamin $B_{12}$ in the treatment of pernicious anæmia.

Hæmatinics contain iron necessary for the formation of hæmoglobin.

Hæmostatics help in the clotting of blood.

Hypnotics help in the production of sleep.

Sedatives and tranquillizers help to calm the nervous system.

Thymoleptic drugs help to change the mood of the patient in states of depression and anxiety.

All "official" drugs and preparations have Latin names, but it is equally proper and correct to refer to them by the English translation.

(*a*) The Latin name may be derived from the Latin botanical name of the plant from which the drug is obtained, e.g.

Digitalis from *Digitalis purpurea* (the purple foxglove).

(*b*) It may be the Latin equivalent of the ordinary English chemical name, e.g.

*Magnesii sulphas* or sulphate of magnesium (magnesium sulphate).

The medical and nursing professions as a whole are very lax in their terminology, and individuals are so often inconsistent, using perhaps the Latin name for one preparation and the English for another. The modern tendency is to use the English form, at any rate for the newer drugs.

Many prescriptions are, however, written in Latin, often in abbreviated form. It will be observed also that the older drugs are often prescribed in the Imperial and Apothecaries' Measures, whereas the newer synthetic drugs are given in doses measured by the Metric System (page 261).

Two faults to be avoided are:

(*a*) Using verbally, abbreviated expressions such as "Mist. sodii sal.", which is quite correct as a written prescription but which should be spoken of in full as "sodium salicylate mixture".

(*b*) Producing the terrible combination of English and abbreviated Latin which is often heard, e.g. "sodii sal. mixture" or "pot. cit. mixture".

Many of the synthetic drugs are extremely complicated chemical compounds with very long names, the meaning of which is only appreciated by a chemist. In such instances, simpler names are often given, either "officially" or as a trade name by the manufacturer. As a rule the "official" name differs from the trade name as the latter is protected by Law and may only be used by the manufacturer. For example, Aspirin was the trade name for acetylsalicylic acid which was originally owned by Bayer. 'Chloromycetin' is a trade name for chloramphenicol.

## The Legal Control of Drugs

Because many drugs are very powerful poisons if employed in improper doses, and others have dangerous habit-forming properties (see page 146), the manufacture, distribution and care of a number of such drugs are carefully protected by Law.

There are two Acts which deal with drugs:

I. The Dangerous Drugs Act (D.D.A.).
II. The Poisons Act.

(These Acts are supplemented by the Dangerous Drugs Regulations and Poisons Regulations made in connection with the respective Acts.)

Certain details of these Acts and Regulations are of importance to the nurse.

### The Dangerous Drugs Act (D.D.A.)

The object of this Act is to prevent the improper sale of drugs having dangerous habit-forming properties. Under it the following important drugs and most of their preparations are controlled:

Opium.

Morphine. Papaveretum ('Omnopon'). 'Nepenthe'.

Pethidine. Pethilorphan, Methadone (Amidone, 'Physeptone', including *Linctus*), Phenadoxone ('Heptalgin').

Levorphanol ('Dromoran'). 'Proladone'. 'Decolid'.
Cocaine.
Diamorphine.   (Heroin), including *Linctus diamorphinæ*.

N.B.—Heroin can only be manufactured under special licence. Its importation into many countries is forbidden on account of its liability to produce addiction.

Indian hemp *(Cannabis indica)*.

Certain preparations containing only small amounts of the above drugs are exempt from the D.D.A., but nevertheless are controlled by the "Poisons" Act—e.g.:

> *Pulvis ipecacuanhæ et opii* (Dover's powder).
> *Linctus diamorphinæ et scillæ* (B.P.C.).
> *Unguentum gallæ cum opio.*

Among rules governing the handling of these drugs are:

1. They can only be ordered by a doctor.

2. In private practice the doctor must keep a record of all purchases and supplies in a separate register or part of a register for each drug.

He must record the amount of the drug actually issued to patients, but is not bound to record the drugs actually administered to patients by himself or under his personal supervision in his presence.

3. Special rules are applied in hospitals, and although the details may vary in different institutions, certain general principles which must fulfil the law are applicable to all.

(*a*) All drugs controlled by the Act must be kept in a special poison cupboard (which should be marked D.D.A.). This cupboard must be kept locked and the key retained *on the person of* a State Registered Nurse (usually the Sister or senior in charge of the ward), who is entirely responsible for the safe custody of the drugs.

(*b*) Fresh supplies can only be obtained from the Pharmacist on an order signed by a Medical Officer or Ward Sister. The drugs should be checked on arrival by the Ward Sister and some form of written receipt given.

(*c*) A register must be kept with separate sections for each drug. Every dose administered must be recorded together with the date, name of the patient and the amount given. This should be filled in and signed by the person giving the drug.

(*d*) These drugs may only be given on the written instructions of a doctor.

It is advisable also that the following details be carried out, although they do not form part of the actual regulations:

(*a*) Each dose given should be checked by an independent witness who sees the phial from which the drug is taken together with the written order of the doctor.

(*b*) The hospital Pharmacist should inspect and check the dangerous drugs in the wards and compare the stocks with the entries in the Dangerous Drugs Register at regular intervals.

(*c*) While it is not possible to mark conspicuously the small phials containing hypodermic tablets, all bottles containing other preparations should be marked with a red D.D.A. label.

(*d*) Sometimes the supply of a dangerous drug, which is not normally part of the ward stock, is ordered for one patient. For example, morphine suppositories, diamorphine linctus or a special mixture containing one of these drugs. In such instances, if the whole supply is not used, the correct procedure is for the nurse in charge to return the surplus personally to the Pharmacist.

## Poisons Act and Rules

In addition to the D.D.A., the care and distribution of a large number of other substances are controlled by Law.

There can be no standard definition of a poison because, clearly, the poisonous effect of any substance depends on the dose given. However, for legal purposes a certain arbitrary standard has been selected and the most dangerous substances are called "Poisons" and are included in the "Poisons List". Not all these substances are necessarily used in medicine but in order that the Regulations can be carried out according to Law they are also classified into a number of Schedules. Schedules 1 and 4 are mainly applicable to medical work.

The Regulations and rules associated with these substances not only concern their sale to members of the public but also to their storage, issue to hospital patients and the methods by which they are labelled.

*Schedule 1* (which includes D.D.A.). The rules state that any of these drugs which are kept in the wards of a hospital must be stored in a cupboard reserved solely for poisons and other dangerous substances. (N.B. Special additional rules apply to D.D.A. drugs.)

*Schedule 4.* For purposes of storage and labelling in hospital this schedule is now divided into the groups 4A and 4B. All drugs in Schedule 4A are included in Schedule 1 and the following rules apply:

The *general public* can only obtain the drugs listed in Schedule 4 on the production of a medical prescription signed by a doctor.

*In hospitals.* (i) These drugs are only supplied to wards from the dispensary on the written order of a Medical Officer or the Sister in charge of the ward.

(ii) The container of the substance must be labelled with the name of its contents and the more powerful poisons (listed in Schedule 1) bear a distinguishing label to indicate that they must be kept in a poison cupboard, specially reserved for such drugs.

(iii) Poison cupboards must be kept locked and must be inspected by the Pharmacist at regular intervals.

(iv) Drugs for internal administration which are listed in the poison Schedules should be kept separate from preparations intended for external use.

*Out-patients.* (i) These drugs are only supplied on the written order of the doctor.

(ii) A record of the issue must be kept for two years on a case paper or card stating the name and address of the patient, the name or initials of the prescriber, the date and amount of the poison supplied.

(iii) The container must be labelled with the name of the hospital supplying it. If it is a lotion, liniment or other medicament for external application, it must be marked "The Liniment" (or appropriate title), "For external use only".

Special poison bottles of characteristic shape which can be recognized by touch (e.g. having vertical ridges and grooves) must be used.

*Schedule 4B.* These drugs are not listed in Schedule 1 and are not subject to the special stringent regulations applicable to this schedule. They must, however, be labelled "Poison" or "Caution" such as "It is dangerous to exceed the stated dose", but they may be stored with other medicines if necessary.

The D.D.A. and Schedule drugs are appropriately noted in the National Formulary and only a few examples are given.

### Schedule 4

In addition to the drugs controlled by the D.D.A., most alkaloids and other powerful poisons (except in certain specified weak dilutions) are included, e.g.

| | |
|---|---|
| Aconite | Amidopyrine |
| Apomorphine | Antimony preparations |
| Atropine and belladonna | Some arsenical preparations |
| Codeine, 'DF 118' | Barbiturates |
| Curare | Carbachol |
| Emetine | Digitalis preparations |
| Ergot alkaloids | Some mercury preparations |
| Hyoscine and hyoscyamine | Mersalyl, 'Neptal' |
| Ouabain | Nalorphine |
| Strychnine and nux vomica | Nitrogen mustard |
| Strophanthin | Phenylbutazone |

### Schedule 4A

As already mentioned all the drugs in this list are included in Schedule 1, e.g.

Barbiturates and preparations containing them
Phenylbutazone

### Schedule 4B

This schedule covers the sulphonamides, tranquillizers, œstrogens, amphetamine, chlorpromazine, methyl pentynol ('Oblivon'), reserpine, hypoglycæmic agents such as chlorpropamide ('Diabinese') and many other drugs.

# CHAPTER 2

# PHARMACEUTICAL PREPARATIONS

There are a number of preparations in use some of which are only occasionally encountered.

## Applicationes or Applications

These are various preparations which are applied to the surface of the body:

e.g. Benzyl benzoate application (*applicatio benzylis benzoatis*)
Dicophane (D.D.T.) application (*Applicatio dicophani*)

## Aquæ or Medicated waters

These usually contain some volatile substance or oil in solution. A number of them are used as flavouring agents.

e.g. Chloroform water (*Aqua chloroformi*).
Peppermint water (*Aqua menthæ piperitæ*).

## Auristillæ or Ear-drops

e.g. Phenol ear-drops (*Auristillæ phenolis*) (page 41).
Spirit ear-drops (*Auristillæ spiritus*).

## Capsulæ amylaceæ or Cachets

These are composed of two discs made of rice flour, the edges of which adhere when moistened. The drug is placed between the discs before sealing. When the whole cachet is moistened it becomes soft and is easily swallowed, it is therefore especially useful for giving a powdered drug.

## Capsulæ or Capsules

These are containers usually made of gelatin. Cachets and capsules are generally used for unpleasant drugs and are intended to be swallowed like pills.

e.g. Vitamin capsules (*Capsulæ vitaminorum*).
Quinalbarbitone capsules (*Capsulæ quinalbarbitoni*), 'Seconal'.

"Spansules" are special proprietary capsules designed to give a regulated, slow release of the drugs they contain.

## Cataplasmata or Poultices

These are soft, pasty external applications used to provide heat and moisture to an inflamed or painful part.

e.g. Kaolin poultice (*Cataplasma kaolini*), 'Antiphlogistine'.

## Collodia or Collodions

These are substances dissolved in a volatile and highly inflammable solvent which evaporates when applied to the surface of the body, leaving a film-like skin or protective covering.

e.g. Flexible collodion (*Collodium flexile*).

### Collunaria or Nasal douches—see page 121.

### Collutoria or Mouth washes—see page 61.

### Collyria or Eye lotions.

## Confectiones or Confections

Jam-like preparations in which drugs are mixed with sugar, syrup or honey are known by this name.

e.g. Confection of senna (*Confectio sennæ*).

## Conspersi or Dusting-powders

These are applied locally to the skin.

e.g. Talc dusting-powder (*Conspersus talci borici*).
Dicophane (D.D.T.) dusting-powder (*Conspersus dicophani*).

## Elixiria or Elixirs

Elixirs are sweet liquid preparations containing syrup, glycerin and, sometimes, alcohol to which various drugs are added. They are very pleasant but rather expensive.

e.g. Elixir of cascara sagrada (*Elixir cascaræ sagradæ*).

## Emplastra or Plasters

Plasters consist of medical substances mixed with lead soap, oil, rubber or resin, and spread on coarse muslin or similar material. They adhere to the skin at body temperature and are usually warmed slightly before application. They are mostly employed as counter-irritants, but may produce blistering on sensitive skins.

e.g. Belladonna plaster (*Emplastrum belladonnæ*).

## Emulsiones or Emulsions

There are many substances which will not normally mix together, such as oil and water, but which may be combined by the addition of a third substance called an emulsifying agent. In an emulsion the globules of fat or oil, instead of running together, remain separate. In some cases the oil and water tend to separate into layers on standing, in spite of the presence of an emulsifying agent, but will re-form an emulsion on shaking. Acacia gum and tragacanth are common emulsifying agents. Milk is an excellent example of a natural emulsion.

e.g. Liquid paraffin emulsion (*Emulsio paraffini liquidi*).

## Extracta or Extracts

By the concentration of various vegetable or animal materials either a solid (*Extractum siccum*) or a liquid extract (*Extractum liquidum*) can be made. The liquid extracts are used in the preparation of medicines given in mixture form, while solid extracts are used for pills and tablets.

e.g. Extract of belladonna (*Extractum belladonnæ*).
Extract of cascara sagrada (*Extractum cascaræ sagradæ*).
Dry extract of opium (*Extractum opii siccum*).

## Enemata or Enemas (see also page 76)

Strictly speaking, an enema consists of the rectal injection of a small quantity of fluid and does not include the administration of large infusions of saline or glucose. Enemas may be classified in the following way:

1. *Those to be returned.*
    Aperient or evacuant: warm water, olive oil, soap, glycerin, turpentine.
2. *Those to be retained.*
    Sedative: starch, starch and opium.

## Glycerina or Glycerins

These are solutions of various substances in glycerin which, being sticky, has the property of adhering to mucous membranes. They may be used in the treatment of affections of the mouth and throat.

e.g. Glycerin of tannic acid (*Glycerinum acidi tannici*).
Glycerin of borax (*Glycerinum boracis*).
Glycerin of phenol (*Glycerinum phenolis*).

## Gargarismata or Gargles

These are fluid preparations used for gargling and are generally similar to or identical with mouth washes.

## Guttæ pro oculis or Eye-drops (page 210)

The drops which are applied to the eye are called guttæ.
e.g. Atropine sulphate eye-drops (*Guttæ atropinæ sulphatis*).
Sulphacetamide eye-drops. (*Guttæ sulphacetamidi*).

## Haustus or Draughts

Drugs in mixture form which are intended to be administered as a single dose are often called draughts.

The administration of a single dose distinguishes them from mixtures, which are usually intended for repeated doses at regular intervals.

### Infusa or Infusions

These are watery solutions containing the active principles of various vegetable drugs. The making of tea is an example of the method of preparing an infusion.

e.g. Fresh infusion of senna (*Infusum sennæ recens*).

## Inhalationes (Vapores) or Inhalations

These are solutions of antiseptic or aromatic drugs or drugs themselves which are volatile or become volatile when poured into hot water.

e.g. Cresote, pine oil, menthol, and Friar's balsam (*Tinctura benzoini composita*) are often used as inhalants.

Anæsthetics such as chloroform, ether and nitrous oxide gas and drugs like amyl nitrite are also given by inhalation.

## Injectiones or Injections

These are sterile solutions of drugs, generally in water but sometimes in oil or other media. They are intended for subcutaneous, intramuscular and, sometimes, intravenous administration.

e.g. Mersalyl injection (*Injectio mersalyli*), intramuscular.
Morphine injection (*Injectio morphinæ*), subcutaneous.

In its wide sense the term injection includes:
1. Intradermal (into the skin).
2. Hypodermic or subcutaneous.
3. Intramuscular.
4. Intravenous.
5. Intrathecal (into the subarachnoid space).
6. Also rectal, vaginal and urethral injections.

N.B. Almost all subcutaneous injections may also be given intramuscularly but not vice versa.

## Insufflationes or Insufflations

These are fine powders blown by a special insufflator directly on to the skin, the mucous membrane of the nose or throat or a wound.

## Lamellæ or Discs

These are very thin, flat wafers made of glycerin and gelatin containing certain drugs which are usually placed in the conjunctival sac of the lower eyelid by means of a camel-hair brush.

e.g. Atropine discs (*Lamellæ atropinæ*).
Cocaine discs (*Lamellæ cocainæ*).
Homatropine discs (*Lamellæ homatropinæ*).

## Lincti or Linctuses (see also page 117)

A linctus is a syrupy or viscous preparation used to allay coughing. The usual dose is 4 to 8 ml. (60 to 120 minims).

e.g. Codeine linctus (*Linctus codeinæ*).
Opiate squill linctus (*Linctus scillæ opiatus*).

## Linimenta or Liniments

The term embrocation is also used to describe the oily soapy or spirituous preparations which are applied to or rubbed into the skin and have a counter-irritant action. They must be labelled "For external use only" and are generally supplied in bottles of characteristic shape and colour so that the risk of giving them internally by mistake is reduced.

e.g. Camphor liniment (*Linimentum camphoræ*, known also as Camphorated oil).

Soap liniment (*Linimentum saponis*).

Methyl salicylate liniment (*Linimentum methylis salicylatis*).

## Liquores or Solutions

These are solutions of chemical substances (rather than animal or vegetable preparations, cf. Extracta).

e.g. Arsenical solution (*Liquor arsenicalis*).

Weak solution of iodine (*Liquor iodi mitis*).

## Lotiones or Lotions

Lotions are watery or alcoholic solutions of drugs for external application to the skin or mucous membranes. They are generally applied on lint or similar fabric, but may be used as washes (see also Collunaria, Collutoria and Collyria).

e.g. Calamine lotion (*Lotio calaminæ*).

Boric acid lotion (*Lotio acidi borici*).

Lead lotion (*Lotio plumbi*).

## Misturæ or Mixtures

The mixture is one of the most common methods of administering medicines by mouth. Mixtures are liquid preparations of one or more drugs, generally flavoured and made up with water to a standard dose of either half or one fluid ounce. They are usually supplied in bottles containing 4 to 20 fluid ounces. The actual composition of standard mixtures varies somewhat in different hospitals and may be altered at will by the doctor to contain the desired dose of the component drugs. The constituents are not fully dissolved in every case and, therefore, the bottle must always be carefully shaken before administration.

e.g. Magnesium trisilicate mixture (*Mistura magnesii trisilicatis*).

Potassium citrate mixture (*Mistura potassii citratis*).

Compound senna mixture (*Mistura sennæ composita*, Black draught).

### Mucilagines or Mucilages

These are viscous aqueous solutions of gums used for the suspension of insoluble drugs.

e.g. Mucilage of acacia (*Mucilago acaciæ*).

Mucilage of tragacanth (*Mucilago tragacanthæ*).

## Nebulæ or Nasal Spray solutions

These are aqueous, oily, glycerinated or alcoholic solutions of drugs intended to be sprayed on the skin or mucous membranes by means of an atomizer. They are generally used as a form of inhalant.

e.g. Ephedrine spray (*Nebula ephedrinæ aquosa*).

Menthol spray (*Nebula mentholis*).

Compound pine oil spray (*Nebula pini composita*).

## Oculenta or Eye ointments

Eye ointments are generally weaker than those applied to other surfaces and contain special drugs of value in eye conditions. They should be applied to the conjunctiva of the lower lid from special tubes or on a sterile glass rod.

e.g. Atropine eye ointment (*Oculentum atropinæ*)

Mercuric oxide eye ointment (*Oculentum hydrargyri oxidi flavum*, Golden ointment).

Penicillin eye ointment (*Oculentum penicillini*).

## Olea or Oils

With the exception of liquid paraffin, which is a mineral oil, and the fish-liver oils, the oils are obtained by distillation or expression from vegetable substances.

e.g. Almond oil (*Oleum amygdalæ*).
  Peanut oil (*Oleum arachis*).
  Oil of clove (*Oleum caryophylli*).
  Linseed oil (*Oleum lini*).
  Olive oil (*Oleum olivæ*).
  Castor oil (*Oleum ricini*).

## Pastæ or Pastes

These are preparations similar to ointments but often having a starchy or glycerin basis. They are generally stiffer and more solid than ointments and their ingredients are, therefore, less easily absorbed. They help to absorb secretions and are not easily rubbed off.

e.g. Starch paste (*Pasta amyli*).
  Zinc and gelatin paste (*Pasta gelatini zinci*), Unna's paste.
  Coal tar paste (*Pasta picis carbonis*).

## Pastilli or Pastilles

These are sweet-like preparations which should be dissolved slowly in the mouth.

## Pessi or Pessaries

A pessary is a cone-shaped mass containing a medicament for introduction into the vagina. It is usually made of cacao butter (oil of theobroma) or gelatin base, which remains solid at atmospheric temperature but is melted by the heat of the body. e.g. Lactic acid pessary (*Pessus acidi lactici*). Acetarsol pessary (*Pessus acetarsolis*).

Buginaria (nasal bougies) and Cereoli (urethral bougies) are pencil-shaped structures of similar composition.

## Pigmenta or Paints

These are liquid preparations applied to the skin or mucous membranes by means of a brush. They are often antiseptic in action. e.g. Iodine compound paint (*Pigmentum iodi compositum*, Mandl's paint).
Others are caustic:

e.g. Chromic acid paint (*Pigmentum acidi chromici*).
Some are used as adhesive varnishes:

e.g. Iodoform compound paint (*Pigmentum iodoformi compositum*, Whitehead's varnish).

## Pilulæ or Pills

Pills are solid spherical bodies containing medicinal agents intended to be swallowed whole and later to dissolve in the alimentary tract. They may be coated with sugar, gelatin or varnish to hide any disagreeable taste.

e.g. Aloes pill (*Pilula aloes*).
Compound rhubarb pill (*Pilula rhei composita*).

## Pulveres or Powders

These are mixtures of finely powdered drugs for internal use when they are usually dispensed in folded paper or capsules. A very small dose of a drug is difficult to handle in powder form and in such cases the bulk of the powder is made up of some other inert substance.

e.g. Compound effervescing powder (*Pulvis effervescens compositus*, Seidlitz powder).
Ipecacuanha and opium powder (*Pulvis ipecacuanhæ et opii*, Dover's powder). This is now usually made as a tablet for convenience.

## Solvellæ or Solution-tablets

These are compressed tablets intended to be dissolved in water to make up solutions. Tablets of a given dosage dissolved in an appropriate amount of water make up solutions of standard strength.

e.g. Mercury iodide solution-tablets (*Solvellæ hydrargyri iodidi*, Biniodide tablets).
Mercury perchloride solution-tablets (*Solvellæ hydrargyri perchloridi*).

## Spiritus or Spirits

Spirits are alcoholic solutions of oils or volatile substances which are only slightly soluble in water.

e.g. Aromatic spirit of ammonia (*Spiritus ammonii aromaticus*, Sal volatile).

## Suppositoria or Suppositories

These are conical solid bodies, not unlike pessaries, containing drugs in a basis of cacao butter (oil of theobroma) or gelatin for insertion into the rectum.

e.g. Glycerin suppository (*Suppositorium glycerini*).
Morphine suppository (*Suppositorium morphinæ*).
Bisacodyl suppository (*Suppositorium bisacodyli*), 'Dulcolax'.

## Syrupi or Syrups

These are fluid preparations of drugs in solutions of sugar.

e.g. Syrup of orange (*Syrupus aurantii*).
Syrup of chloral (*Syrupus chloralis*).
Compound syrup of figs (*Syrupus ficorum compositus*).
Syrup of iron phosphate with quinine and strychnine (*Syrupus ferri phosphatis cum quinina et strychnina*, Easton's syrup).
Compound syrup of iron phosphate (*Syrupus ferri phosphatis compositus*, Parrish's Food).

## Tabellæ (Tablettæ) or Tablets

Tablets consist of drugs compressed in a mould. Many drugs intended to be dissolved in sterile water for hypodermic injection are supplied in tablet form. As a general rule tablets to be taken by mouth should be crushed before administration and given with a draught of water. Some tablets, e.g. *Tabellæ glycerylis trinitratis* (page 94) are allowed to dissolve under the tongue.

e.g. Acetysalicylic acid tablets (*Tabellæ acidi acetyl salicylici*, Aspirin tablets).

## Tincturæ or Tinctures

These are solutions of crude drugs in alcohol and resemble spirits but differ from them in their mode of preparation. Their individual doses differ considerably.

e.g. Tincture of belladonna (*Tinctura belladonnæ*).
Compound tincture of benzoin (*Tinctura benzoini composita*, Friar's balsam).

Tincture of digitalis (*Tinctura digitalis*).
Tincture of nux vomica (*Tinctura nucis vomicæ*).
Tincture of stramonium (*Tinctura stramonii*).

## Trochisci or Lozenges

These are solid flat tablets containing drugs incorporated in a gum or sugar basis. They dissolve slowly and are intended to be sucked. They usually have an astringent or antiseptic action on the mucous membrane of the mouth and throat.

e.g. Liquorice lozenges (*Trochiscis glycyrrhizæ*, Brompton lozenges).

Benzocaine compound lozenges (*Trochisci benzocainæ compositi*).

## Unguenta or Ointments

Ointments are semi-solid preparations containing drugs mixed with materials such as soft paraffin ('Vaseline'), lard, wool fat or Lanette wax. They are intended to be spread on or rubbed into the skin.

e.g. Boric acid ointment (*Unguentum acidi borici*).

Ammoniated mercury ointment (*Unguentum hydrargyri ammoniatum*).

Creams are similar to ointments but contain water and an emulsifying agent. Their ingredients are more penetrating and more easily absorbed than from greasy ointments.

e.g. Calamine cream (*Cremor calamini*).

Zinc oxide cream (*Cremor zinci oxidi*).

## Vapores or Vapours

These are similar to inhalations.

**Vaccines** and **sera**—see page 241.

# CHAPTER 3

# THE ADMINISTRATION OF DRUGS

Therapeutic substances are administered or applied in a number of different ways.

## 1. Via the alimentary tract

   (*a*) By the mouth (per os)

| | |
|---|---|
| Capsules | Mixtures containing: |
| Draughts | Extracts |
| Elixirs | Mucilages |
| Linctuses | Oils |
| Lozenges | Solid drugs |
| Pastilles | Solutions (liquores) |
| Pills | Spirits |
| Powders | Tinctures |
| Tablets | Waters (aquæ) |

   (*b*) By the rectum (per rectum)

| | |
|---|---|
| Enemas | Suppositories |

## 2. Via the respiratory tract

Inhalations including anæsthetics

| | |
|---|---|
| Sprays | Vapours |

## 3. Via the uro-genital tract

   (*a*) By the urethra (per urethram)

| | |
|---|---|
| Bougies | Injections |

   (*b*) By the vagina (per vaginam)

| | |
|---|---|
| Douches | Pessaries |

## 4. Drugs applied to the skin

   (*a*) Local applications.

| | | |
|---|---|---|
| Collodions | Glycerins | Paints |
| Creams | Liniments | Pastes |
| Dusting powders | Lotions | Plasters |
| Fomentations | Ointments | |

(*b*) Baths.

(*c*) Ionization.

## 5. Drugs applied to mucous membranes

Many of the above may also be applied to mucous membranes. In addition:

(*a*) Mucous membrane of the mouth.

| | |
|---|---|
| Gargles | Mouth washes (collutoria) |
| Lozenges | Pastilles |

(*b*) Mucous membrane of the nose.

| | |
|---|---|
| Inhalations | Nasal douches (collunaria) |
| Insufflations | Sprays |

(*c*) The eye.

| | |
|---|---|
| Eye discs (lamellæ) | Eye ointments (oculenta) |
| Eye drops (guttæ) | Eye washes (collyria) |

(*d*) The ear.

| | |
|---|---|
| Ear drops (auristillæ) | Insufflations |

## 6. Drugs given by injection

(*a*) Intradermal (into the skin).

> e.g. B.C.G. Vaccine
> Tuberculin tests, e.g. Mantoux
> Schick test for diphtheria

(*b*) Hypodermic or subcutaneous. (Into the loose tissue spaces just beneath the skin.)

> e.g. Narcotic drugs such as morphine
> Stimulant drugs such as nikethamide

(*c*) Intramuscular or into a muscle. e.g. Mersalyl.

(*d*) Intravenous or into a vein. e.g. 'Ferrivenin'.

(*e*) Intrathecal or into the spinal canal.

> e.g. Penicillin, streptomycin
> Spinal anæsthetics

The term "parenteral" means "not through the alimentary canal" and is used to imply some type of injection.

### Technique of Administration

### Rules for the oral administration of drugs

The administration of drugs is a matter of great importance to the nurse and is one of the routine duties which carries with it great responsibility.

Many drugs are powerful poisons; while doses of others are carefully calculated in order to produce the desired effect.

Absolute accuracy of measurement in every case is essential and is an important part in a nurse's training. Familiarity should never lead to carelessness. In the event of any doubt entering the nurse's mind about the correctness of a dose or the drug she is about to give, there must be no hesitation in referring the matter to a senior officer.

Points to remember about administering medicines are:

1. Punctuality, with special regard to the instructions before and after meals and special directions e.g. "with water".

(Medicines so ordered should be given 20 minutes before meals or immediately after meals.)

2. Read the label on the bottle and check the drug and dose with the patient's treatment card.

3. Make a habit of shaking the bottle in each case, irrespective of whether the medicine is clear or containing a sediment. This should be done by inverting the bottle several times, with the forefinger on the cork to prevent accidental spilling.

4. Measure the dose carefully into a suitable medicine measure. A special measure should be used for doses under 8 ml. (120 minims, 2 drachms). The measure should, if possible, be read while standing on a flat surface. If not, it must be held at eye level, taking care not to tilt the measure either backwards or forwards, a movement which will obviously produce an inaccurate reading.

It is not a wise practice to rely on the marking often found on medicine bottles and is certainly bad training.

5. Hold the cork with the little finger while pouring out.

6. Give the medicine or tablet to the patient immediately and watch him take it.

It is the proud boast of some patients that they pour all their medicine down the sink. Do not leave drugs lying about or permit unauthorized persons to handle them. In a private house circumstances may, of course, modify this procedure.

7. Observe and report any signs of over-dose, reaction or

intolerance. In this connection, if any mistake should unfortunately be made in the administration of a drug either by giving the wrong drug or dose, the nurse must immediately report the fact, irrespective of any possible consequences to herself. An error reported at once can sometimes be rectified without serious consequences to the patient.

8. Have all hypodermic injections and dangerous drugs checked by a second person and enter the dose given in the poison register when this is required.

9. Try to make the administration of unpleasant drugs as agreeable as possible, e.g. give iron mixtures with a straw to prevent blackening of the teeth, and give the patient an opportunity of brushing the teeth without delay. Sweets, fruit juice, a mouth-wash or a piece of bread may help to remove a disagreeable taste.

10. Keep medicine bottles clean by wiping after use and always pour out of the side away from the label, i.e. keep the label uppermost.

11. Remember that tablets and capsules are supplied in various strengths and, therefore the labelled dose must be carefully checked with the treatment card.

## Notes on the administration of drugs

*Linctus:* Should be sipped slowly.

*Lozenge* and *pastille:* Should be sucked slowly.

*Mixture:* See that the patient takes any sediment which tends to collect in the medicine glass.

*Pill, capsule:* Should be given with a drink of water and swallowed whole.

*Cachet:* Should be soaked in water before swallowing.

*Oil:* Occasionally two or three drops of a volatile oil, such as oil of peppermint, are ordered for flatulence and are best given on a cube of sugar.

Olive oil, arachis oil and liquid paraffin are given by mouth in the usual way, using a porcelain measure or oil cup.

Many cunning devices have been thought of for disguising the taste of the old favourite, castor oil (*Oleum ricini*), e.g.

(i) Adding 60 minims (4 ml.) of compound tincture of cardamom to each half ounce.

(ii) Giving the oil in capsules.

(iii) Warm the oil cup, put in a small amount of whisky, brandy, lemon or orange juice, then the oil, and finally float a thin layer of the flavouring agent on top. Follow with a small piece of bread.

(iv) Castor oil mixture (*Mistura olei ricini*, B.P.C.) is an emulsion flavoured with orange flower and cinnamon waters.

*Suppository:* This should be inserted into the rectum with the patient in the lateral position. It may be dipped in warm water (the purpose being to melt the surface of the suppository) to facilitate introduction, which should be carried out slowly with the gloved finger, taking care to pass the suppository through the anal sphincter into the rectum.

*Bougie:* Dip in warm oil or water before insertion.

*Pessary:* Slight moistening may be necessary before insertion, but usually there is sufficient mucous secretion present to make introduction easy.

*Powder:* (i) The contents of a paper may be placed on the back of the patient's tongue and followed by a drink of milk or water.

(ii) Sprinkle on the surface of a little milk.

(iii) Mix with jam in a sandwich for children.

(iv) Effervescent powders should be stirred in half a tumbler of water and taken at once, e.g. Seidlitz powder.

*Tablet:* As a rule a tablet should be crushed, placed on the back of the tongue and swallowed with a draught of water.

Tablets of glyceryl trinitrate and isoprenaline should be allowed to dissolve under the tongue i.e. sublingually.

Tablets of potassium chlorate and antacid tablets (e.g. 'Gelusil') should be allowed to dissolve slowly in the mouth.

*Tincture:* Occasionally a tincture is ordered to be given as such, e.g. tincture of digitalis. The dose should be measured accurately, using a minim measure. Minims should *not* be estimated by counting a number of drops.

## The Action of Drugs

It will be clear from consideration of the enormous number of drugs at our disposal and the divers conditions for which they may be employed, that no very precise summary can be given of their mode of action. However, among the ways in which drugs can act are:

1. The direct action on micro-organisms and parasites on the surface of the body or on other objects.

   e.g. The use of antiseptics for sterilizing instruments or as lotions applied externally; benzyl benzoate emulsion applied for scabies.

2. By giving drugs which have a direct lethal effect on organisms within the tissues of the body.

   e.g. (a) The use of chemotherapy (sulphonamides etc.) and antibiotics, such as penicillin, against bacteria which are sensitive to their action.

   (b) Mepacrine for malaria.

3. By producing some direct and obvious chemical effect.

   e.g. (a) Neutralizing the hydrochloric acid in the gastric juice by giving antacids such as magnesium trisilicate or aluminium hydroxide.

   (b) Turning an acid urine alkaline by giving citrate; or an alkaline urine acid with acid sodium phosphate.

4. Producing the desired effect by some definite physiological action which can be clearly explained by a knowledge of the actual processes which normally occur.

   e.g. Atropine paralyses the nerve-endings to the muscle of the pupil of the eye and its administration results in dilatation of the pupil. On the other hand, physostigmine (eserine) stimulates the nerve-endings and its action is opposite to that of atropine, for it causes the pupil to contract.

The action of digitalis on the conducting tissues of the heart in the bundle of His, whereby it blocks a number of the frequent and irregular impulses coming from the auricle (atrium) in auricular fibrillation, is also a good example.

5. Drugs may be given to replace some missing factor which should normally be supplied by the body. Such drugs

are usually chemically identical with the missing substance and are either made in the laboratory or obtained from some suitable animal.

e.g. (a) Insulin to supply the missing pancreatic hormone in diabetes. Various ductless gland preparations e.g. thyroid, pituitary and ovarian extracts.

(b) Vitamin $B_{12}$ or liver to supply the missing extrinsic factor in pernicious anæmia.

6. Vitamins, and drugs like iron and calcium given to supply dietetic deficiencies. Iron and calcium may also be required when their absorption is defective.

7. Many other examples might be given, but they will become apparent as individual drugs are considered.

A *placebo* is a medicine given to please or satisfy a patient without having any special pharmacological effect. It is really, therefore, a form of psychotherapy.

### Idiosyncrasy

Idiosyncrasy may be defined as an abnormal or unusual response to a normal dose of a drug. (The word is derived from the Greek: *idios* = one's own, *syncrasis* = blending.) It is a form of over-sensitivity which is closely allied to allergy: in fact, the term "drug allergy" is sometimes used.

It is only met with in isolated cases but, in such instances, an ordinary dose may produce toxic symptoms which are unpleasant, alarming or even dangerous. There is no known explanation of this abnormal sensitivity and the symptoms manifested are frequently similar to those seen when an overdose of the drug has been taken by a normal person.

The symptoms may appear immediately, particularly after injections, but may be delayed for some hours or even days.

Since the nurse may administer the drug herself or the patient will be under her observation after it has been given, the subject is clearly one of great importance to her. Any unusual symptoms occurring after a drug has been taken should, therefore, be reported without delay. The condition may develop after a drug has been given internally, but not infrequently external applications to the skin produce severe local reactions. Sometimes a patient is aware of the sensitivity and gives information on the subject beforehand.

The most common types of reaction which occur are:

1. Rashes and skin eruptions.

2. General symptoms including collapse, nausea, vomiting and giddiness.

3. Agranulocytosis, due to an unexpected toxic action of the drug in the bone marrow. This is a serious condition which may prove fatal (see page 103).

While it is difficult to exclude any particular drugs, the following are important:

1. *Quinine*, causing deafness, giddiness, headache, nausea, shivering, noises in the head, disturbances of vision and transient rashes such as urticaria or erythema.

2. *Sodium salicylate and aspirin*, causing noises in the head (tinnitus), deafness, malaise, nausea, rapid pulse or an erythematous rash.

N.B.—Aspirin occasionally causes hæmatemesis or melæna, and may also produce serious reactions in asthmatics.

3. *Potassium iodide*, causing increased secretion from the respiratory tract resembling a severe cold in the head, laryngitis and skin eruptions similar to acne. Iodine given internally in other forms may produce the same effects (iodism).

4. *Bromides.* Skin eruptions such as pustular acne or erythema are the most common manifestations. Mental dullness and general weakness may also be present. The symptoms of bromism resemble iodism and there may be an increase in the mucous secretion from the respiratory tract.

5. *Calomel.* An ordinary dose may produce symptoms of severe collapse in some individuals.

6. *Cocaine* (including procaine, 'Novocain', etc.). Malaise, vomiting, pyrexia; collapse with pallor, rapid pulse and slow respirations, and sometimes convulsions or fits, may all occur. Death occasionally follows from respiratory paralysis.

7. *Sulphonamides.* Drugs of this group may produce serious symptoms in some individuals, e.g. changes in the white cells

of the blood (agranulocytosis), hæmaturia, pyrexia after the initial lesion for which the drug has been given has subsided (drug fever), and skin rashes. (See page 228.)

8. *Penicillin* sometimes causes rashes or even severe collapse in sensitive persons, and streptomycin may also give rise to troublesome eruptions in those who handle it.

### Tolerance

This may be of two types: (i) *Natural* tolerance, which is really the direct opposite of idiosyncrasy and implies that the individual resists the action of a certain drug and can tolerate much larger doses than a normal person. (ii) *Acquired.* This means a state induced in the normal person by the prolonged use of a drug whereby he can gradually tolerate increasing doses which would, if administered in the first place, have produced toxic symptoms.

Tolerance is a common phenomenon and is exhibited by a number of drugs. Tobacco and alcohol are obvious examples. The first cigarette may produce nausea, vomiting and a greenish pallor of the skin, while a seasoned smoker may consume up to fifty cigarettes a day without any obvious symptoms. The difference in effect between two persons consuming the same amount of alcohol is also well known.

Among the important drugs used in therapeutics for which tolerance may be acquired are: opium and morphine, atropine and belladonna, stramonium and arsenic. (Page 157.)

It must always be remembered however, that when a drug is discontinued the acquired tolerance is usually lost and, if the drug is re-commenced at a later date, ordinary doses must be used.

It is not known what acquired tolerance depends on. It may be that some chemical "anti-body" is formed or that the tissues fail to absorb the drug fully. In some cases the excretion may be more rapid, in others the drug is more quickly destroyed or converted into some inert substance.

### Drug addiction

This is a state in which the individual acquires a craving for a particular drug, often to such an extent that life becomes unbearable without it. Not only psychological upsets but also physical disturbances such as palpitation and sweating may occur if the patient is deprived of the drug. In addition to those drugs referred to in the Dangerous Drugs Act (page 6) patients may become addicted to alcohol, paraldehyde, dexamphetamine and many other substances.

## Cumulative effect

When a drug is taken one of two things may happen.

(a) It may be destroyed or converted into some inert or inactive substance by the tissues, especially the liver.

(b) It may be excreted unchanged by the kidneys, bowel, lungs or skin.

Clearly there will be a definite relationship for each drug, between the rate at which it is taken in and the rate of its destruction or excretion and, as a rule, the dosage and intervals at which any drug is administered are adjusted to meet this situation. It follows that if the rate of administration is greater than the rate of destruction or excretion, the drug will accumulate in the tissues and increase in amount with each dose taken.

Some drugs are especially liable to show this phenomenon and will produce the symptoms of overdosage or poisoning.

Digitalis is an important example. Mercury, arsenic and lead are others. In lead poisoning, small quantities of lead may be absorbed into the body over a long period and, finally, when a certain concentration exists in the tissues the typical symptoms appear, e.g. colic and various types of paralysis.

### Dosage according to Age

The "official" dose of the majority of drugs is calculated for their administration to an adult of average weight. It is quite clear that much smaller doses will be required for children and infants and that, roughly speaking, these will be dependent upon the age and size of the child.

Various formulæ have been devised in order to calculate the doses required by children, e.g. according to *Young's Formula*, the dose for children less than 12 years of age may be obtained by dividing the age, by the age plus twelve. Thus for a child of 6:

$$6 \div (6 + 12) = \tfrac{1}{3}$$

Therefore $\tfrac{1}{3}$ of the "official" adult dose would be given.

There are other factors also to be considered. Children tolerate the following drugs well, and relative larger doses than those obtained by the application of the above formula can be given with safety:

Aperients.                                   Arsenic.
Atropine and belladonna.      Hyoscyamus.

On the other hand, it is most important to remember that the following are badly tolerated and much smaller doses must be used:

Morphine, opium and other narcotics.

In old age too it is usually advisable to reduce the average dose somewhat.

The following table is of value, but in all cases experience in the use of drugs is the most important factor.

### DOSES PROPORTIONATE TO AGE

| AGE | | DOSE |
|---|---|---|
| 1 month | | $\tfrac{1}{20}$ of adult dose |
| 3 to 6 months | | $\tfrac{1}{15}$ to $\tfrac{1}{12}$ ,, ,, |
| 9 to 12 ,, | | $\tfrac{1}{12}$ to $\tfrac{1}{10}$ ,, ,, |
| 1 to 2 years | | $\tfrac{1}{10}$ to $\tfrac{1}{8}$ ,, ,, |
| 2 to 4 ,, | | $\tfrac{1}{8}$ to $\tfrac{1}{6}$ ,, ,, |
| 4 to 6 ,, | | $\tfrac{1}{6}$ to $\tfrac{1}{4}$ ,, ,, |
| 6 to 8 ,, | | $\tfrac{1}{4}$ to $\tfrac{1}{3}$ ,, ,, |
| 8 to 12 ,, | | $\tfrac{1}{3}$ to $\tfrac{1}{2}$ ,, ,, |
| 12 to 14 ,, | | $\tfrac{1}{2}$ to $\tfrac{2}{3}$ ,, ,, |
| 14 to 18 ,, | | $\tfrac{2}{3}$ to $\tfrac{3}{4}$ ,, ,, |
| 18 to 60 ,, | | 1 ,, ,, |
| 60 to 90 ,, | | $\tfrac{3}{4}$ to $\tfrac{2}{3}$ ,, ,, |

# CHAPTER 4

# DISINFECTANTS AND ANTISEPTICS

Only a section of the large subject of sterilization falls within the province of Materia Medica, namely, the killing of bacteria by chemical methods. This presents three problems:

1. The killing of bacteria away from the human body, viz. the sterilization of instruments, utensils, linen, dressings, excreta, etc.

2. The killing of bacteria on the surface of the body and in wounds.

3. The killing of bacteria within the tissues of the body by drugs given by internal administration. (See Chemotherapy, antibiotics, etc.)

## Methods of sterilization

The following methods of killing or removing bacteria may be employed:

### I. *Physical methods*

(*a*) *Heat.* (1) Ordinary boiling for periods up to 20 minutes depending on the nature of the article. Two minutes boiling kills most bacteria, but spores are not necessarily destroyed by the most prolonged boiling.

The addition of 2 per cent washing soda to the water is more lethal to the bacteria and spores.

(2) Steam under pressure, as produced in the autoclave.

(3) Dry heat which is not so effective as moist heat and, in comparison, requires to be of a higher temperature and to act for longer periods.

(*b*) *Radiation.* Direct exposure to sunlight or ultra-violet rays is effective in destroying a number of organisms.

(*c*) *Filtration.* It is possible to remove bacteria from water and other fluids by passing them through a special very fine

B *                          33

filter of the Berkefeld or Pasteur-Chamberland type. Viruses are smaller than ordinary bacteria and will pass through such filters, hence the term "filter-passing virus" is sometimes used.

## II. Chemical methods

The majority of these drugs owe their germicidal or antiseptic action to one of the following properties:

1. The power to extract water from the bodies of bacteria.
2. The power of coagulating proteins.
3. A general poisonous action on protein.
4. The liberation of oxygen.

The value of soap and detergents as aids to disinfection should not be overlooked. Most of them have no germicidal power in themselves but, when used on the hands or other articles, very efficiently remove the superficial layer of grease in which bacteria are lodged, and so facilitate the subsequent application of germicides. Very few disinfectant substances can be combined with toilet soap and the majority of the "carbolic soaps" are useless from a germicidal point of view. On the other hand, Lysol, a solution of cresol in soap, is a powerful germicide. The detergent cetrimide ('Cetavlon') has mild antiseptic properties.

Whenever possible, sterilization of instruments and utensils by boiling is to be preferred to chemical methods, while the autoclave is indispensable for dressings and gloves.

The main uses for chemical disinfectants in this connection are to keep sterile instruments free from further contamination; in emergency when other methods are not available and for non-boilable appliances, e.g. gum-elastic catheters and some electrical connections.

Some form of local application is the only method of attempting to render the skin aseptic. Careful washing with soap and water or cleaning with a detergent such as cetrimide ('Cetavlon'), followed by a suitable germicide, e.g. tincture of iodine, acriflavine, etc., is reasonably successful.

The disinfection of lavatories and drains is practically impossible and most disinfectant fluids poured down them only act as deodorants.

## Disinfectants and Antiseptics

Strictly speaking, an antiseptic is a substance which prevents the growth of micro-organisms but does not necessarily kill them, so that their growth may be possible after the removal of the drug. Such action is sometimes described as *bacteriostatic*. A disinfectant or germicide kills bacteria and, by comparison with antiseptics, may be called *bactericidal*. All disinfectants are, therefore, antiseptics, but an antiseptic is not necessarily a germicide.

It must be remembered, however, that a substance in strong concentration may be germicidal, but in weaker solutions may only act as an antiseptic, so that no exact distinction can be made between the two terms.

The following is a summary of some of the important factors upon which disinfectant and antiseptic action depends:

1. The strength of the disinfectant.

2. The time for which it acts.

3. The temperature.

4. The nature of the material in which it has to act. The presence of pus or other organic matter retards the action of some drugs of this class.

5. The type of the infecting organisms.

*1. The strength of the disinfectant.* It has just been mentioned that a substance in strong concentration may be bactericidal but in weaker solutions may only act as an antiseptic, i.e. as a bacteriostatic.

This is a most important fact to realize, for many of the drugs of this group are used in various strengths for different purposes, and dilution affects each disinfectant to a markedly different degree.

Thus, phenol in concentrated form acts very rapidly, in dilutions up to 1 in 100 it acts with reasonable rapidity but in solutions weaker than this is almost ineffective and organisms will survive for many hours in a strength of 1 in 150. In other words the phenol in a "Carbolic bath", formerly given at the end of an infectious illness, was quite useless.

*2. The time of action.* Speaking generally, this varies

with the concentration of the drug. The stronger the solution of the drug, the shorter the time required to kill bacteria.

The dyes, mercury salts and the salts of other metals tend to be slow in action, whereas disinfectants dependent upon the liberation of chlorine are relatively rapid.

*3. Temperature.* The action of disinfectants is, in most instances, increased to some extent by a rise in temperature. Therefore, preparations for external use should be employed at body temperature whenever possible.

*4. The nature of the material.* This specially applies to the presence of pus, blood and other organic matter, such as necrotic tissue, which tend to decrease the activity of many antiseptics and germicides.

*5. The type of the infecting organism.* The most powerful disinfectants are germicidal to all organisms. On the other hand, some disinfectants, as well as the more powerful ones in weaker concentrations, show what may be called "selective action". That is, a disinfectant may be more effective against one organism than another.

For example, staphylococci are very susceptible to gentian violet dye. Dyes of the flavine group are more active against streptococci than staphylococci. These facts are of particular importance in the dressing and irrigation of wounds.

## Important Disinfectants and Antiseptics

Much research has been carried out on disinfectants. The great difficulty has been to produce those which can be used not only outside the body but also on the human tissues, because so many substances which are lethal to bacteria also injure the tissues and are, therefore, of no value in disinfecting the skin or irrigating wounds, for they will do more harm than good.

The ideal requirements for a disinfectant are:

1. To be strongly lethal to bacteria but non-injurious to human tissues (i.e. non-toxic and non-corrosive).

2. To be easily soluble in water, saline and serum, and to act efficiently in the presence of pus, blood or dead tissue.

3. To be inexpensive.

The disinfectants and antiseptics most commonly used can be classified roughly into several main groups:

1. Acids and alkalis.
2. Solutions of certain metallic salts.
3. Various organic compounds (including alcohols and coal-tar products, etc.).
4. The halogens.
5. Oxidizing agents.
6. Dyes. (a) Aniline type. (b) Flavine type.
7. Various other substances.

## 1. Acids and Alkalis

Strong mineral acids (such as nitric, sulphuric and hydro-chloric acids) and alkalis (caustic potash and caustic soda) are corrosive and destroy all living matter. They also dissolve or damage many substances in common use. They are, therefore, unsuitable for application as disinfectants either to the surface of the body or on utensils in concentrated form.

They are, however, occasionally employed as caustics (i.e. to burn away tissue), for example, the application of strong nitric acid to warts.

In appropriate dilution they are sometimes employed in treatment. It will be recalled that the gastric juice contains hydrochloric acid (0·2 per cent) and that this is sometimes referred to as the "antiseptic barrier" of the stomach. Dilute hydrochloric acid, 10 per cent (*Acidum hydrochloricum dilutum*, B.P., dose up to 4 ml. (60 minims)) is occasionally given in dyspeptic conditions and in some cases of pernicious anæmia, a disease in which hydrochloric acid is absent from the gastric juice.

There are a number of other weak acids not belonging to the mineral acid group which are non-corrosive and used in therapeutics for other purposes. The majority are given internally and are considered later. Others are employed externally for various purposes. The following are some which are given internally:

Acetysalicylic acid (aspirin).    Lactic acid.
Ascorbic acid (Vitamin C).    Mandelic acid.
Citric acid.    Nicotinic acid.

Lactic acid is also used as an antiseptic in vaginal douches and pessaries.

Tannic acid was once used as an external application on account of its astringent properties and its power of tanning or coagulating proteins on an open surface, e.g. for burns.

### Boric acid (*Acidum boricum*)

Boric acid, a white crystalline substance, is an antiseptic of feeble action which is non-irritant. It has the power of inhibiting growth of many organisms and is used for a number of purposes.

As a lotion, the strength of which may vary from 1 to 4 per cent, it is used for irrigating the eye, ear, nose, vagina or bladder.

Many dusting powders used in the treatment of skin diseases, such as eczema, contain boric acid, and it may also be employed in ointments.

It was formerly used as a preservative for food, but this is now illegal.

### Salicylic acid (*Acidum salicylicum*)

This occurs as colourless crystals and has some antiseptic properties, especially against fungi. For this purpose it is used in ointments in certain skin diseases, e.g. *Unguentum acidi salicylici compositum* (Whitfield's ointment). It is also used in foot-powders. In plasters (*Emplastrum salicylicum*) or collodion, it is used for corns and warts.

Salicylic acid is not given internally, but its derivatives, sodium salicylate and acetylsalicylic acid (aspirin) are well known (see page 153).

### Acetic acid (*Acidum aceticum*)

This is an organic acid which is present in vinegar. Its only possible use as an antiseptic lies in the fact that a 2 per cent solution is an effective dressing for infections due to *Bacillus pyocyaneus* (a good example of selective action previously mentioned). 'Phenoxetol' is a more effective preparation for this purpose.

## 2. Solutions of certain metallic salts

The metallic salts which can act as disinfectants are those which have the power of coagulating proteins, such as silver nitrate, copper sulphate, zinc sulphate, biniodide and perchloride of mercury.

### Silver nitrate (*Argenti nitras*)

This substance has special uses and may be employed in solid form or as a solution.

(*a*) In solid form it is used as a caustic (lunar caustic) to destroy excess of granulation tissue in an open wound or callous ulcer. The stick is slightly moistened and rubbed lightly on the area of granulation tissue, care being taken to avoid contaminating the surrounding skin. This process may be painful and produces a white appearance, which later turns black. When thus applied it destroys all the tissues and organisms with which it comes in contact. It has also been used to cauterize dog bites with a view to preventing rabies, a disease transmitted by the bite of a rabid dog.

N.B.—Silver nitrate stains on the skin may be removed by mercuric chloride solution.

(*b*) As a solution for irrigating the bladder in chronic cystitis the strength may be gradually increased from 1 in 10,000 to 1 in 2000.

(*c*) For eye drops and as a prophylactic against ophthalmia neonatorum in a new-born infant, a less irritating colloidal silver preparation such as *Guttae argentoproteini* ('Argyrol' 10 per cent), in which silver is combined with a protein, has been used.

**Copper sulphate** (*Cupri sulphas*)

Copper sulphate is used in Benedict's test for glycosuria.

**Zinc sulphate** (*Zinci sulphas*)

This substance, and also zinc chloride, is occasionally used in the form of antiseptic eye drops.

**Mercury biniodide** (*Hydrargyri iodum rubrum* or Red mercuric iodide)

This is a very poisonous antiseptic which is used externally. It may be employed in aqueous or spirituous solutions, viz.:

Aqueous solution—1 in 2000 to 1 in 5000 for application to wounds.

1 in 5000 to 1 in 10,000 as a vaginal douche.

Spirituous solution—1 in 500 to 1 in 2000 to render the skin aseptic.

It is wise to wash out wounds or the vagina after its use with sterile water in order to prevent the risk of poisoning from the absorption of mercury.

**Mercury perchloride** (*Hydrargyri perchloridum*, Mercuric chloride, Corrosive sublimate)

This is a colourless, poisonous, antiseptic which must not be confused with mercurous chloride (calomel). Solutions of it and mercury biniodide may be artificially coloured to minimize the risk of being mistaken for water or other harmless liquid. Its solution is used in strengths up to 1 in 1000 for external purposes, but it should not be applied to steel instruments on account of its action on the metal.

Both mercury biniodide and perchloride are undoubtedly bacteriostatic, but their bactericidal powers are uncertain. They tend to be slow in their action, which is further retarded by the presence of blood.

N.B.—Some skins are sensitive to mercury and its use may result in dermatitis.

### 3. Various organic compounds

**The alcohols**

Chemically there are a number of different alcohols but only two require special mention, viz.:

Ethyl alcohol.
Methyl alcohol.

*Ethyl alcohol.* In its pure form and when free from any trace of water it is referred to as absolute alcohol.

Ethyl alcohol has maximum antiseptic properties as a 70 per cent solution, but in stronger or weaker concentrations is less effective. It is useful for rendering the unbroken skin aseptic, but it is painful when applied to raw surfaces and this, together with the fact that the presence of proteins reduce its activity, renders it unsuitable for application to wounds. Applied externally, however, alcohol hardens the skin and is useful in preventing bedsores. It evaporates quickly and is used in cooling lotions in the treatment of sprains and contusions. It is the type of alcohol present in fermented beverages (page 220) and is also the basis of a number of pharmaceutical preparations, e.g. tinctures and some liniments.

Surgical spirit is a purer form which can only be purchased from a chemist on a prescription.

*Methyl alcohol.* This is present in methylated spirit. It is a very toxic substance and may cause blindness when taken by mouth. Ordinary methylated spirit is an impure preparation which is artificially coloured violet.

Methylated spirit is inflammable and is sometimes used for the purpose of "flaming" bowls, etc., with a view to sterilizing them. This, however, is a most uncertain and dangerous method which should only be resorted to in emergency when no other means are available. There is never any excuse for its use in hospital.

## The coal-tar disinfectants

A large number of chemical substances are produced from coal tar. Many have germicidal properties and a number of others have various medicinal uses. Among the most important of the former are phenol (carbolic acid) and the cresols, which are the basis of the disinfectants of the lysol type.

### Phenol (*Acidum carbolicum*)

Pure phenol is a caustic which occurs in colourless crystals and has a characteristic pungent odour, but it is rarely used in this state.

Phenol is most commonly supplied in the form of a lotion (1 in 20), which may be further diluted for special purposes. It should not be employed as a dressing for open wounds as its absorption may either damage the tissues locally or cause general toxic symptoms.

A stronger solution (1 in 20) is used for disinfecting excreta in typhoid fever and similar conditions.

Liquefied phenol (*Acidum carbolicum liquidum*) contains 80 per cent phenol and is sometimes used as a caustic. It must not be confused with *Lotio phenolis* (referred to above, which is usually of 1 in 20 strength).

Phenol is sometimes dissolved in glycerin instead of water. Solutions in glycerin are much less caustic (and of lower germicidal power) than those in water. Thus glycerin and phenol ear-drops (*Auristillæ phenolis*) contain 7·5 per cent of phenol but under no circumstances should these be diluted with water which will render them caustic in action. It follows that the ear must be carefully dried after syringing with lotions before glycerin and phenol drops are instilled.

Phenol also has some local anæsthetic action, hence its value as a mouth-wash or gargle (*Gargarisma phenolis*) in painful affections of the mouth and throat, for which it is also employed as a lozenge. As ear-drops it is, therefore, of value both on account of its antiseptic and anæsthetic properties.

Other preparations include:

Glycerin of phenol (*Glycerinum phenolis*, 16 per cent).
Phenol ointment (*Unguentum phenolis*, 3 per cent).

It must be emphasized that the correct modern term for this drug is PHENOL and that carbolic acid, no longer the "official" name, should be dropped.

**Lysol** (*Liquor cresolis saponatus*, B.P.—Solution of cresol with soap)

Lysol is a solution of cresol in soap. It is a powerful disinfectant and caustic. It may be employed undiluted for sterilizing instruments, which should be immersed for 5 minutes. Care should always be taken to avoid splashing the skin and especially the eyes, and it should be applied to utensils with a mop or by using rubber gloves. Utensils should then be rinsed with sterile water before use. Splashes of phenol or lysol on the skin should be immediately removed by swabbing with glycerin or olive oil. Water must be avoided.

Weaker solutions are also germicidal, but must be allowed to operate for longer periods.

It should not be employed on the skin in concentrations exceeding 2 per cent. For douches, a 1 per cent solution is generally employed (60 minims to the pint is convenient but is slightly less than 1 per cent).

'Sudol' is a non-caustic proprietary form of lysol.

There are many proprietary preparations similar to lysol which are used for the same purposes, but in strengths appropriate for each, e.g. 'Izal' and 'Jeyes' Fluid'.

Chloroxylenol solution (*Liquor chloroxylenolis*, 'Roxenol') may be used (*a*) for cuts, 1 in 80, or 4 ml. (60 minims) to $\frac{1}{2}$ pint of water, (*b*) vaginal douche, 1 in 40, or ½ oz. to 1 pint of water, (*c*) mouth wash, 1 in 480 to 1 in 160, or 1 to 2 ml. (10 to 30 minims) in ½ pint.

'Dettol'. This is a proprietary disinfectant similar to chloro-xylenol which is specially effective against streptococci. It has the advantage of being non-irritant and non-toxic even in con-centrated form. A dilution of 1 in 10 is generally recommended for application to the skin. It may be used as a liquid, oint-ment or cream.

**Chlorhexidine** ('Hibitane'). This is an important, non-irritating synthetic disinfectant which remains active in the presence of blood and body fluids and, therefore, has many uses.

It is prepared as a 5 per cent solution or concentrate and also as a powder, obstetric cream (1%), antiseptic cream (1%) and lozenge. It may be mixed with the detergent, cetrimide, to form a very useful cleansing agent.

**Hexachlorophene** ('Phisohex') may be used for pre-operative skin cleansing, routine hand washing and skin care generally.

**Dequalinium** ('Dequadin') has antiseptic properties and is used in lozenges, pessaries, paint, cream and impregnated gauze.

### 4. The halogens

The term halogen (which is derived from two Greek words meaning "salt producer") is used to include the elements chlorine and iodine (and bromine), because their salts are found in sea-water. The disinfectant drugs of this group owe their germicidal power to the liberation of chlorine or iodine in small quantities.

**Chlorine** itself is a poisonous, intensely irritating, green gas which has no medicinal use in this form. The following compounds are, however, employed:

Chlorinated lime or bleaching powder (*Calx chlorinata*).
Hypochlorite solutions, which include Eusol, 'Milton' and Dakin's solution.
The chloramines.

Chlorinated lime or bleaching powder is a disinfectant and deodorant of special use in disinfecting fæces, deodorizing drains and lavatories, and is the basis of other preparations.

Eusol (*Liquor calcis chlorinatæ cum acido borico*) is a solution of chlorinated lime and boric acid which is used for the irrigation and dressing of wounds. It is non-irritating and non-toxic. Solutions tend to decompose on keeping and should not be more than three weeks old. Dressings are applied in the form of gauze soaked in Eusol and should not be covered with waterproof material.

Dakin's solution (*Liquor sodii chlorinatæ chirurgicalis*) is of similar composition and has the same uses.

'Milton' is a pleasant proprietary preparation having sodium hypochlorite as a base which may be used for cleaning and irrigating wounds, as a dressing and for storing dentures.

Chloramine is a complicated organic compound containing chlorine and has similar uses to the former preparations.

Chlorine preparations are also used in the disinfection of drinking water and the water in public swimming baths. The unpleasant taste of the water may be neutralized by the addition of sodium thiosulphate (photographic "hypo") after the chlorine has been permitted to act for a definite period.

### Iodine (*Iodum*)

Iodine is an element which is in the form of bluish-black crystals. It is intensely irritating to the skin, which it stains a deep reddish brown. This may be removed by solutions of alkali or sodium thiosulphate.

In addition to its antiseptic properties, iodine and its salts have many other uses in medicine.

The disinfectant preparation most commonly employed is tincture of iodine (*Liquor iodi mitis*, B.P.—Weak solution of iodine, $2\frac{1}{2}$ per cent). This is an alcoholic solution which must be distinguished from *Liquor iodi aquosus*, B.P.C., sometimes known as Lugol's iodine. The latter is used for internal administration, especially in cases of thyrotoxicosis before operation, in doses increasing from 2 to 10 minims (see also page 193).

Tincture of iodine is employed as a skin disinfectant and sometimes as a vaginal douche (60 minims, 4 ml., to the pint). It may also be used as a counter-irritant over painful areas, for example, in dry pleurisy. For this purpose a stronger preparation, *Liquor iodi fortis* (containing 10 per cent iodine) is occasionally employed.

Preparations: (*a*) for external use.

   Strong solution of iodine (*Liquor iodi fortis*).

   Weak solution, or tincture, of iodine (*Liquor iodi mitis*).

   Compound iodine paint, or Mandl's paint (*Pigmentum iodi compositum*). (Sometimes used for sore throats.)

   Iodine ointment (*Unguentum iodi*).

(*b*) for internal use.

   Aqueous solution of iodine or Lugol's iodine (*Liquor iodi aquosus*).

*Radio-active iodine* ($I^{131}$) is used in the diagnosis and treatment of disorders of the thyroid gland.

## Iodine compounds for X-ray diagnosis

There are a number of substances containing iodine which are opaque to X-rays and which can be introduced into the body without causing harm. They can be used for outlining the bronchial tree (bronchogram), the uterus (uterogram), the fallopian tubes (salpingogram), the spinal cord (myelogram), the gall bladder (cholecystogram), the urinary tract (pyelogram).

In the case of the cholecystogram the dye is taken by mouth and is excreted by the liver so that normally it fills the gall bladder. A pyelogram may be obtained by injecting the dye intravenously.

These compounds include:

1. Iodized oil (*Oleum iodisatum*) or 'Lipiodol,' which is used for bronchograms, uterograms and salpingograms.

2. Diodone injection, which is used for intravenous and retrograde pyelograms and also for other radiographic procedures, is available in various concentrations and is also obtainable under proprietary names viz.

35 per cent, 'Arteriodone', 'Perabrodil', 'Aridone'.

50 per cent, 'Perabrodil forte'.

70 per cent, 'Vasidone'.

'Pyelosil' is prepared in all strengths. It may also be employed for outlining blood vessels (arteriography).

3. Iodoxyl ('Uropac') and 'Hypaque' are also used for intravenous pyelography.

4. 'Myodil' which may be injected intrathecally by means of lumbar puncture.

5. Gall bladder dyes which include iodophthalein, 'Opacol', Pheniodol and 'Telepaque' which are given by mouth and 'Biligrafin' given intravenously.

**Iodoform.** This is an organic compound, yellow in colour, with a strong odour which many persons find objectionable. It has the reputation of being an antiseptic, but its value is doubtful. It is sometimes used as a powder for insufflation into the ear. Mixed with bismuth subnitrate in the form of a paste (*Pasta bismuthi et iodoformi*, known also as B.I.P.P.), it is sometimes used for packing wounds and sinuses.

Whitehead's varnish (*Pigmentum iodoformi compositum*) may be employed to protect the skin from irritating discharges.

N.B.—Some individuals are sensitive to iodine in any form. Toxic effects such as flushing, nausea, vomiting, skin eruptions and, rarely, collapse may be observed.

## 5. *Oxidizing agents*

The most important drugs which owe their antiseptic properties to the liberation of oxygen in the presence of organic matter are hydrogen peroxide and potassium permanganate.

### Hydrogen peroxide (*Hydrogenii peroxidum*, $H_2O_2$)

This is used in the form of a solution (*Liquor hydrogenii peroxidi*) which contains about 3 per cent of hydrogen peroxide but is described as "10 volumes". This means that it can liberate 10 times its volume of oxygen, and a stronger solution of double this strength is described as being of "20 volumes".

In the presence of organic matter or pus, bubbles of oxygen are liberated, and this has a valuable mechanical action in removing discharges from wounds in addition to its antiseptic property. It must be used with care in the irrigation of deep cavities, especially the thorax, and there must be a free outlet for drainage since the oxygen liberated may produce dangerous distension unless it can escape.

Hydrogen peroxide is used as a mouth-wash and has a slightly bitter taste. After its use as ear-drops the meatus should be carefully dried by swabbing or its epithelium will become sodden. It also acts as an astringent and is a good hæmostatic. It is used for bleaching fabrics and the hair, the latter being turned an easily recognizable, un-natural yellow colour not comparable in beauty with that of the natural blonde. It forms the basis of 'Sanitas'.

## Potassium permanganate (*Potassii permanganas*)

This occurs in the form of dark purple crystals. It is a disinfectant and deodorant and owes its power to the fact that in solution it gives off oxygen in the presence of organic matter. As it does so it turns brown, an indication that the solution has lost its efficiency. Permanganates form the basis of Condy's Fluid.

It is used in strengths of 1 in 5000 for application to wounds, ulcers, etc., and 1 in 10,000 as a vaginal douche, gargle and mouth-wash. The solid is sometimes applied to snake-bites. Permanganate stains in fabrics may be removed by applying sulphurous acid and then washing in water.

Preparations:

> Solution of potassium permanganate (*Liquor potassii permanganatis*, 0·1 per cent).
> Potassium permanganate gargle (*Gargarisma potassii permanganatis*, 0·025 per cent).

### 6. Dyes

The most important germicidal dyes can be divided into two main groups which may be conveniently called (*a*) the aniline group and (*b*) the flavine group, thereby indicating their general chemical type.

## (a) Dyes of the aniline group

Their main use is in disinfecting the skin and in the anti-septic treatment of wounds. Their action is relatively slow and, as has already been pointed out, is selective in character; that is, they only have a marked effect on certain organisms.

The most important dyes of this group are **gentian violet** (crystal violet) and **brilliant green**. The green and violet dyes are sometimes used in combination in the form of Bonney's blue (*Liquor tinctorium*). They are most effective against staphylococci and are more useful in preventing infection than in the treatment of established sepsis, although they are of value in some cases of impetigo. Solutions may be either aqueous or spirituous. For application to the skin a 1 per cent solution is employed; for wounds, dilutions of 1 in 1000 to 1 in 2000 are used.

With acriflavine, they form the basis of triple dye jelly which is used as a tanning compound in the treatment of burns.

Gentian violet capsules have been given internally for the treatment of thread worms.

Other dyes of this group employed for different purposes include:

| | |
|---|---|
| Congo red. | Methylene blue. |
| Indigo carmine. | Scarlet red. |

**Indigo carmine,** when given by intramuscular injection, is excreted by the kidneys and is used as a test of renal efficiency. The principle is to observe the rate at which the dye is excreted from each kidney after ureteric catheterization.

**Methylene blue** is also used as a test of renal efficiency.

## (b) Dyes of the flavine group

These dyes are yellow in colour and show marked selective action against streptococci. The three most commonly used are **acriflavine, proflavine** and **Acramine Red.** They are used both for application to the skin and for irrigating wounds. As distinct from many other germicides, their action is not decreased by the presence of blood and they do not interfere with the phagocytic power of the leucocytes. They are generally employed in strengths of 1 in 1000, but they must not be mixed with Eusol, Dakin's solution, lysol or mercurial solutions. Stains are removed with dilute hydrochloric acid.

Emulsions in liquid paraffin are also frequently used, but their antiseptic power is thereby considerably reduced.

### 7. *Other substances*

Among the other disinfectants which have not so far been mentioned, the most important is formaldehyde.

### Formaldehyde (*Formaldehydum*)

Formaldehyde itself is a pungent gas which irritates the eyes and mucous membranes of the respiratory tract. It is used in the form of a solution, *Liquor formaldehydi* (formalin), which contains about 40 per cent of the pure substance. This is a powerful disinfectant but, in a solution of this strength, is unsuitable for application to the skin. It is useful for spraying the walls and furniture of infected rooms, and special fumigators for the liberation of the gas are employed to fumigate rooms. The room is sealed for 3 to 4 hours.

Formaldehyde has an important use in the sterilization of catheters which are exposed in a special box to its vapour. The vapour is obtained either from *Liquor formaldehydi* or from tablets of paraform, which must not be confused with the formalin tablets for internal administration.

Mouth washes, gargles and tablets are also available and are weaker preparations.

In conclusion, the utmost care must be taken in the use of antiseptics and disinfectants. When employed they must be used in the appropriate strength and allowed to act for the correct time. So many are available that no one can be expected to know the details of all, but it should be regarded as a duty to be familiar with those in common use.

Although these drugs are valuable, remember that unless correctly used they can afford a very dangerous false sense of security. Do not imagine for one moment that dipping the hands in a bowl of highly coloured liquid (reputed to be an antiseptic but probably inactive in the dilution employed) by the side of the typhoid or other infectious patient has any other value than to remind you to go and wash your hands at once, and properly, with soap and water. In any case, you should have been wearing rubber gloves!

## Deodorants

Deodorants or deodorizers may be defined as substances which are used to destroy or remove disagreeable odours. Many of them are also disinfectants or antiseptics and have been mentioned in this connection. They may be used to get rid of odours from drains or from offensive discharges from wounds. For the former purpose, chlorinated lime and Jeyes' Fluid are examples of the most economical.

For wounds, hydrogen peroxide, 'Sanitas', Eusol and potassium permanganate are all useful or charcoal may be applied as a powder.

Drugs of the lysol and phenol types act as deodorants. Offensive smells can also to some extent be covered by the pungent odour of iodoform or by the burning of special deodorizing cones.

Special electrical apparatus which produces ozone is an efficient method of deodorizing a room. An "Airwick" is also useful.

A number of deodorant sprays with fancy names are available which, by their own potency, effectively mask unpleasant odours.

Chlorophyll tablets taken by mouth are claimed to deodorize the breath.

Cetrimide ('Cetavlon') is a detergent which also has antiseptic properties (see page 55).

# CHAPTER 5

# DRUGS ACTING ON THE SURFACE OF THE BODY

There are a number of specialized forms of treatment which are used in various skin conditions and also for the relief of superficial pain viz.:

Radiation: *X*-rays, radium, ultra-violet light.

Heat:   (*a*)  cautery
        (*b*)  radiant heat, infra-red rays

Cold:   (*a*)  carbon dioxide snow (for warts and nævi)
        (*b*)  evaporating lotions

In addition, medicaments may be employed by local application in various forms including:

Lotions and liniments.

Ointments, creams and pastes.

Paints, powders and poultices.

In order that the above may be applied to the skin a number of different bases or vehicles are employed to incorporate the medicaments used. These include:

1. Powders consisting either of unmixed powdered drugs or containing starch, which absorbs moisture, or talc or fuller's earth which does not.

2. Water: (*a*) Soluble substances may be dissolved in water and applied in various strengths which are usually expressed as a percentage solution.

(*b*) "Shake lotions", such as calamine lotion, in which the substance does not dissolve but after application the water evaporates leaving the dried medicament in powder form on the skin surface.

3. Alcohol: This is included in some lotions for the cooling effect which occurs with rapid evaporation. It is also used as a vehicle in some solutions, liniments and paints, e.g. Tincture of iodine which has an antiseptic action.

4. Water-soluble vehicles and emulsifying agents: These are non-oily substances of complicated chemical structure

(including glycols and stearates) which produce emulsions from which medicaments are easily absorbed. They include Macrogols and substances such as lanette wax which assist in the mixture of watery and oily substances.

5. Oily and greasy vehicles: These include soft and hard paraffin, also wool fat and the wood alcohols derived from it. They form the basis of ointments.

The majority of drugs used can be classified according to their main actions:

## Antiseptic applications

Some of the antiseptic or bacteriocidal substances already mentioned in the previous chapters are suitable for external application in the form of lotions, paints or creams etc. Among them are:

Salicylic acid and mercuric chloride lotion (B.P.C.).

Formaldehyde (3 per cent) lotion.

Copper and zinc sulphate lotion (astringent and mildly antiseptic).

Brilliant green and crystal violet paints.

Cetrimide cream.

Chlortetracycline cream.

Proflavine cream.

Ammoniated mercury ointment.

Boric acid ointment.

Ointments containing penicillin, streptomycin or sulphon-amides carry a high risk of causing sensitization and are, therefore, contraindicated as local applications. Tetracycline, chloramphenicol and neomycin are less risky. Impetigo and local skin fissures are the types of condition treated in this way.

## Antiparasitic preparations

These include benzyl benzoate application used in the treatment of scabies. Croamiton cream may also be used in this condition. Sulphur ointment, although effective, is liable to cause further dermatitis.

Gamma benzene application ('Lorexane'), medicated lethane oil and dicophane application are used for pediculosis of the head. Oil of sassafras is now rarely employed. Blue ointment (*Unguentum hydrargyri dilutum*, B.P.) may be used for the treatment of body lice. Dicophane or 'D.D.T.' (dichlor-diphenyl-trichlorethane) is an insecticide which has many medical and domestic uses.

*Fungicides.* There are numerous fungus infections of the skin, hair and nails, including ringworm and monilia infections. Local applications used in treatment of conditions such as "athlete's foot" include magenta paint, benzoic acid compound (Whitfield's) ointment and zinc undecenoate ointment. Proprietary preparations include 'Mycil' (chlorphenesin) and 'Asterol'.

Griseofulvin is a rather expensive oral antibiotic used in ringworm and certain other fungus infections. The average adult dose is 1 gram daily for three to six weeks. Finger-nail infections may require longer treatment.

## Antipruritics

Itching may be a symptom both of skin disorders and general disease such as diabetes, jaundice, drug intoxication and anxiety states. Lotions and creams such as phenol, calamine, croamiton ('Eurax') have a local action. Antihistamine drugs by mouth may be helpful but when applied locally may cause sensitization.

Local steroid preparations such as hydrocortisone and prednisolone lotions and creams (up to 1 per cent) are valuable and may be combined with antibiotics such as tetracycline in infective skin lesions.

## Caustics (Escharotics)

A caustic is a substance which has a burning or destructive action on living tissue. Many concentrated disinfectants are caustics and have been mentioned already. They include:

Strong nitric, hydrochloric and sulphuric acids.
Glacial acetic acid and trichloracetic acid.
Chromic acid.
Acid mercuric nitrate.
Silver nitrate, copper sulphate and zinc chloride.
Caustic potash and caustic soda.

Strong acids are sometimes used to destroy warts.

Silver nitrate is used to burn down excess of granulation tissue in a healing wound, in order that the epithelium may have an opportunity of growing over the surface of the granulation tissue from the sides of the wound. Silver nitrate is also applied to dog-bites.

Copper sulphate is applied to the inner surface of the eyelids in trachoma.

Acid mercury nitrate in solution, may be applied to the skin lesions in lupus.

Chromic acid, 25 per cent, is sometimes applied as a cauterizing agent to the septum of the nose to stop hæmorrhage from a bleeding-point in severe epistaxis.

### Emollients

Emollients are bland oily substances applied to the skin or mucous membranes to protect them from irritation or to render them soft. They are therefore useful in the treatment of abrasions, chapped hands and healing surfaces. They also serve as vehicles for other drugs applied for various skin diseases in the form of ointments. (Not all ointments, however, are emollient in action.) The most important emollients are:

Wool fat and 'Lanolin'.          Soft paraffin ('Vaseline').
Olive oil.                               Castor oil.
Arachis oil.

*Barrier Creams* are preparations designed to protect the skin against irritant substances which may be encountered by industrial workers or nurses. They may also be used to protect the skin of patients from discharges. Silicone barrier creams are water-repellant and are used against water-soluble irritants. They are useful in the prevention of napkin rash and in the treatment of bed sores.

### Demulcents

These are substances similar to emollients which are applied to mucous membranes and may be given internally. They are used:

For protecting inflamed mucous surfaces, e.g. white of egg or milk given in corrosive poisoning.

Masking the unpleasant taste of certain drugs.

Suspending insoluble drugs.

In addition to the above emollient drugs, white of egg, gelatin, starch, gum and tragacanth are all demulcents.

### Sedative applications

When the skin is acutely inflamed wet dressings are often indicated. These include aluminium acetate lotion, coal tar lotion, lead lotion, calamine lotion and sodium chloride solution (normal saline).

Starch poultices are useful for removing crusts such as may occur in severe impetigo of the scalp.

### Soaps

Soaps are cleansing agents made by combining oils or fats with alkalis. There are three main types:

Curd or animal soap made from animal fat and caustic soda.

Hard soap made from vegetable oils and caustic soda.

Soft soap made from vegetable oils and caustic soda or potash but containing glycerin. Ether soap is a 40% solution of soft soap in alcohol and ether.

Soapless washing powders for domestic use are special (sulphonated) fatty alcohols. An example of this type of compound used medicinally is Liquor Sulphestolis ('Teepol') which is employed as a skin cleanser and shampoo.

### Detergents and cleansing agents

These are cleansing agents for the skin. In addition to the use of ordinary soap and water, ether soap, spirit soap or a detergent when the skin is grimed with oil, it may be necessary to remove dirt or crusts from injured or inflamed skin by using olive-oil, arachis oil or starch poultices.

Detergents are more effective cleansing agents than soap and water and in addition many have antiseptic properties. Among the most important are:

*Cetrimide* ('Cetavlon', C.T.A.B.) which is generally used as a 1% solution. A cream is also available. Napkins may be washed in 1 in 1000 to prevent napkin rash.

Benzalkonium chloride ('Roccal', 'Zephiran') has similar

properties. Various strengths are employed according to the particular requirements.

A number of household detergents and washing powders are in use and are well advertised! These occasionally cause dermatitis in persons with a sensitive skin. Care should always be taken not to employ them in concentrated form, and always to rinse the hands well after use.

## Astringents

These are drugs which check secretion and cause drying of a surface. They are most frequently used on mucous membranes and, therefore, in addition to their application to the mouth and throat, they are also given internally for their action on the bowel, especially in the treatment of diarrhœa.

Calamine lotion and lead lotion have a slightly astringent action and are used in the acute stages of eczema and also to allay irritation in urticaria. Calamine liniment, various creams (e.g. ichthammol), and Lassar's paste are used in the later stages of eczema. Coal-tar preparations have mildly astringent and antiseptic properties.

Other powerful astringents for external use include tannic acid, alum, iron perchloride and weak solutions of silver nitrate and zinc sulphate.

## Stimulating preparations

In order to stimulate the growth of granulation tissue in healing wounds, Red lotion (*Lotio rubra*, containing zinc sulphate) or Scarlet red ointment (*Unguentum rubrum*, containing scarlet red dye) may be applied. Cod-liver oil applied externally has similar properties. Preparations used on the unbroken skin, include ichthammol ointment, zinc and coal tar paste.

## Softening preparations (Keratolytics)

It is sometimes necessary to soften the horny layers of the skin, and for this purpose pastes or ointments containing resorcin or salicylic acid may be used.

Chrysarobin is used for removing the scales of psoriasis.

Dithranol ('Cignolin') has a similar action.

Stains produced by these substances may be removed with a solution of chlorinated lime.

Salicylic acid collodion is used in the treatment of corns.

## Irritants

Depending upon the severity of their action, irritants may be classified as:

1. Rubifacients.    2. Vesicants.    3. Caustics (page 53).

**Rubifacients** are drugs used to produce reddening or mild inflammation of the skin. By their action they cause the blood vessels to dilate so that the part to which they are applied becomes red and hot. For example, ammonia, camphor, menthol, oil of wintergreen (methyl salicylate), turpentine, all of which are employed in the form of liniments, tincture of iodine and belladonna plaster. A poultice containing kaolin ('Antiphlogistine') also has a rubifacient action. It is mainly used for the relief of pain and for local inflammatory lesions such as boils.

**Vesicants** or blistering agents produce an intense irritation resulting in the formation of blisters. They are no longer used, but include croton oil and cantharides (*Liquor epispasticus* contains cantharidin which is a most violent poison).

*Counter-irritation.* Remedies such as the liniments, plasters, poultices and paints already referred to, applied to the surface of the body with the object of relieving pain or congestion in an underlying organ by producing mild inflammation of the skin are called counter-irritants.

Pain resulting from a diseased organ is often felt in some part of the body wall rather than in the organ itself. As examples, the pain of a gastric ulcer may be felt in the epigastric region of the abdominal wall and is associated with excessive tenderness of the skin (hyperæsthesia) in that area. Pain in gall-bladder disease may be felt in the right shoulder.

This phenomenon is called "referred pain" and is due to the fact that the organ affected has a nerve supply from the same segment of the spinal cord as that of the area of skin in which the pain is felt.

## Styptics or Hæmostatics

### Drugs which check bleeding

Styptics are drugs applied *locally* to a bleeding surface

C

with the object of checking hæmorrhage. They are unlikely to be of marked effect except in oozing or capillary hæmorrhage, bleeding from arteries obviously requiring ligature. Most astringents are also styptics,

> e.g. Tannic acid.
> Solution of ferric chloride (*Liquor ferri perchloridi*).
> Silver nitrate.
> Alum.

Hydrogen peroxide has a useful local hæmostatic action. Adrenaline (1 in 1000) applied locally acts by causing the blood-vessels in the bleeding area to contract. Caustics will stop hæmorrhage but are not employed for this purpose.

**Snake venom** obtained from a viper (e.g. 'Stypven') is a very powerful hæmostatic which may be applied on cotton wool in a dilution of 1 in 10,000. It may be used for plugging bleeding tooth sockets and is especially valuable in the control of bleeding in hæmophilia.

The application of absorbable **gelatin sponge** to a bleeding surface promotes a clot which forms rapidly and adheres to the tissues. It may be moistened before use with saline or penicillin solution and a wound closed over it. Complete absorption takes place in four to six weeks. Oxidized cellulose and calcium alginate are similarly employed and may, if necessary, be soaked in a solution of thrombin before use.

The treatment of hæmorrhage is, however, a much wider subject and involves the use of drugs given internally:

1. Morphine is given to allay restlessness and thereby to cause a general lowering of blood pressure.

2. Calcium may be given by mouth (calcium lactate gr. 30, t.d.s.) or by injection in the form of calcium gluconate, with a view to aiding clotting but is of doubtful value.

3. Special hæmostatic preparations have been used, e.g.

> (a) 'Thromboplastin' which consists of a solution of pro-thrombin and thrombokinase.
> (b) 'Coagulen-Ciba', a preparation of blood platelets obtained from the cow.

4. Special drugs such as ergot and ergometrine, and posterior pituitary extract ('Pitocin', page 202) are given to check bleeding from the pregnant uterus because they have a special action on this organ, causing its muscle to contract.

5. In certain circumstances the tendency to excessive bleeding may be checked by the administration of vitamin K (Menaphthone) (page 184). Vitamin K is necessary for the production of prothrombin and is given as a pre-operative measure in cases of jaundice. 'Rutin' is a drug used in cases in which increased fragility of the capillaries is present.

## Drugs which prevent clotting (Anticoagulants)

There are a number of substances which have a directly opposite *local* action to the styptics, namely, they prevent blood from clotting. These include:

1. Sodium and potassium citrates. They act by preventing the activity of the calcium salts present in the blood by combining with them to form inactive compounds. Use is made of this in blood transfusion by collecting blood into 3·8 per cent citrate solution.

2. Sodium oxalate has a similar effect and is used for preventing the clotting of blood taken for certain laboratory tests, e.g. blood cholesterol, creatinine, urea, uric acid and the Van den Burgh and other liver function tests. Sodium fluoride may be used in blood-sugar estimation.

N.B.—Citrates given internally do not have any effect on the clotting of blood. Oxalates and fluorides are poisonous.

3. Contact with oil, grease or paraffin wax.

4. Hirudin, a substance obtained from the leech, delays clotting. This explains why a leech bite continues to bleed for a considerable period.

5. The anti-coagulant drugs given *internally*, including Heparin, phenindione ('Dindevan') and nicoumalone ('Sinthrome'), are considered on page 109.

### Diaphoretics

The sweat glands are situated in the skin all over the body but are most abundant in the axillæ, palms, soles and forehead, and have been estimated to number about two million. They are supplied by the sympathetic nerves.

Drugs which increase the amount of perspiration are called diaphoretics. They may act:

1. By stimulating the sweating centre in the central nervous system.

2. By stimulating the sweat glands.

3. By dilating the cutaneous blood-vessels, which increase the blood-supply to the glands.

It is not always possible to say exactly how and where each diaphoretic drug acts. The following are examples of diaphoretics:

Pilocarpine, a very powerful drug, which stimulates the nerves of the involuntary system supplying the sweat glands.

Alcohol, which acts by dilating the cutaneous blood-vessels.

Ipecacuanha. This has a mild diaphoretic action and is a constituent of Dover's powder (*Pulvis ipecacuanhæ et opii*).

The main use of diaphoretics is to render a feverish patient with a hot dry skin more comfortable. The evaporation of the sweat also tends to cause a fall in the body temperature (i.e. diaphoretics have an antipyretic action).

**Anhydrotics** are drugs which diminish the amount of sweat. The most important are atropine and belladonna, and stramonium. They also cause dryness of the mouth.

### Antipyretics

An antipyretic is a drug which reduces fever. There are a number of antipyretic drugs, but all have other actions for which they are employed, so that their antipyretic effect is incidental to their use for other purposes.

The normal temperature of the body is maintained by a balance between the heat produced and the heat lost, and that this is controlled by the heat-regulating centre in the brain. Heat lost is dependent on (a) the amount of blood circulating in the vessels of the skin and (b) the amount of sweat secreted and the rate of its evaporation.

A drug may therefore have an antipyretic effect:

(i) by acting on the heat-regulating centre.

(ii) by dilating the blood-vessels in the skin.

(iii) by increasing the amount of sweat.

The drugs which have an antipyretic action include:

Aspirin and sodium salicylate.     Phenacetin.     Quinine.
All diaphoretics.

The methods employed when it is desired to lower body temperature are tepid or cold sponging, a tepid bath, etc., details of which are given in books on Nursing.

# CHAPTER 6

# DRUGS ACTING ON THE ALIMENTARY SYSTEM

## DRUGS ACTING ON THE MOUTH AND PHARYNX

Drugs used for their action on the mouth and pharynx are most commonly employed in the form of mouth-washes, gargles, paints or lozenges, which may be demulcent, astringent, antiseptic or sedative in character, e.g.

| | |
|---|---|
| *Demulcent:* | Glycerin. |
| | Glycerin of borax (*Glycerinum boracis*). |
| *Astringent:* | Glycerin of tannic acid. |
| | Solution of iron perchloride (*Liquor ferri perchloridi*). |
| *Antiseptic* | Phenol (0·5 per cent). |
| | Hydrogen peroxide (60 minims to one ounce). |
| | Glycerin of thymol (as in 'Glycothymoline' and *Collutorium thymolis composita*). |
| | Gentian Violet Paint. |
| | Mandl's paint (*Pigmentum iodi compositum*). |
| | Lozenges e.g. 'Dequadin', 'Bradosol', 'Tyrozets'. |
| *Sedative:* | Benzocaine lozenge (*Trochisci benzocainæ compositi*). |
| | Phenol or aspirin gargles, which have an anæsthetic effect. |
| *Steroid:* | Hydrocortisone tablets ('Corlan') for ulcers in the mouth. |

These are generally used in various forms of stomatitis, pharyngitis and tonsillitis.

## DRUGS ACTING ON THE SALIVARY GLANDS

Drugs may be given either to increase (sialogogues) or decrease (anti-sialogogues) the flow of saliva. Drugs may also decrease the flow of saliva and cause dryness of the mouth when given for other purposes. Thus atropine reduces the amount of saliva and this may be a troublesome side-effect of its administration.

Hyoscine and stramonium, sometimes used in large doses in the treatment of paralysis agitans, also produce excessive dryness of the mouth which may be counteracted by giving pilocarpine, a drug which stimulates the flow of saliva.

*Sialogogues* (increasing flow): pilocarpine.

*Anti-sialogogues* (decreasing flow): atropine, hyoscine, stramonium.

## DRUGS ACTING ON THE TEETH AND GUMS

Toothpastes are generally made of slightly abrasive powders, with soap, to which some antiseptic and a flavouring agent may be added.

Toothache due to dental caries may be relieved by inserting into the cavity a pledget of cotton wool soaked in oil of cloves or 'Dentalone', which have a local anæsthetic action.

Various antiseptic astringents, gentian violet or tincture of iodine may be applied to the gums in cases of gingivitis.

## DRUGS ACTING ON THE STOMACH

In order to understand the various actions of drugs on the stomach it is important to recall the main points concerning its physiology.

1. The stomach is a hollow organ consisting of serous, muscular and mucous coats. The muscular coat (having circular, longitudinal and oblique fibres) gives it the power of peristaltic movement. The circular fibres also form the pyloric sphincter which relaxes at intervals to allow partially digested food to enter the duodenum.

The glands of the mucous membrane secrete pepsin, which converts proteins into peptones; hydrochloric acid which acts as an antiseptic barrier and aids the action of pepsin; also rennin and the intrinsic factor essential for the formation or absorption of the anti-anæmic factor (Vitamin $B_{12}$).

Hydrochloric acid may be absent (achlorhydria), diminished (hypochlorhydria) or increased (hyperchlorhydria).

The nerve-supply of the stomach includes nerves passing to

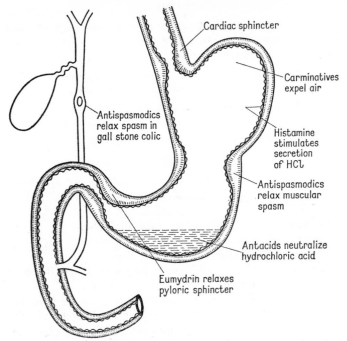

Cardiac sphincter

Carminatives
expel air

Antispasmodics
relax spasm in
gall stone colic

Histamine
stimulates
secretion
of HCl

Antispasmodics
relax muscular
spasm

Antacids neutralize
hydrochloric acid

Eumydrin relaxes
pyloric sphincter

FIG. 1—Diagram illustrating the action of some drugs
on the stomach, etc.

the vomiting centre in the medulla oblongata, which is also
connected to the higher centres of the brain.

Drugs acting on the stomach can be considered according
to whether they act (*a*) on its movements or (*b*) on the mucous
membrane or its secretions, viz.:

1. Carminatives.
2. Emetics.                          Acting on
3. Sedatives and anti-emetics.   (*a*) stomach movements.
4. Stomachics, including bitters. (*b*) the mucous membrane.
5. Antacids.
6. Substitutes.
7. Drugs used in radiography.

## Carminatives

A carminative is a drug which aids the expulsion of wind from the stomach by increasing the tone of its muscle and stimulating its movements, e.g.

   (i) The volatile oils such as oil of peppermint (*Oleum menthæ piperitæ*) 0·2 ml. ($\frac{1}{2}$ to 3 minims).

  (ii) Aromatic spirit of ammonia (*Spiritus ammonii aromaticus* or Sal volatile) 4 ml. (15 to 60 minims) in water.

 (iii) Various preparations of ginger (*Zingiber*).

## Emetics

Emetics are drugs which produce vomiting and are therefore responsible for causing much more violent movements in the stomach muscle than carminatives.

Emetics acting directly on the stomach include:

Tincture of ipecacuanha 30 ml. ($\frac{1}{2}$ to 1 ounce).

Zinc sulphate, 2 grams (10 to 30 grains).

Salt and water $\left.\right\}$ 8 grams (120 grains) in 5 to 8 ounces
Mustard and water of water.

The most important emetic acting directly on the vomiting centre is: Apomorphine 6 mg. ($\frac{1}{10}$ grain) given hypodermically.

N.B.—Excessive doses of many drugs will cause vomiting, and it is common after the administration of sulphonamide drugs, and in digitalis poisoning. In a number of persons the usual doses of morphine appear to stimulate the vomiting centre.

Emetic drugs are not often employed, as in most cases in which it is desired to empty the stomach of its contents it is preferable to wash it out with water or saline after passing a stomach tube. In some circumstances, however, it may be necessary to use them. They may be employed to remove the contents of the stomach when it is over-distended with food. They are of value, as an emergency measure, in some cases of poisoning due to substances other than caustics. There is danger in using them after caustic poisoning because the violent contraction of the organ may cause rupture of its walls if they are severely damaged by the corrosive substance.

Emetics are sometimes of value in children suffering from bronchitis, when the bronchi are full of mucus and there is no effective cough, because the act of vomiting is then often accompanied by the expulsion of mucus from the bronchial tubes.

## The Mechanism of Vomiting

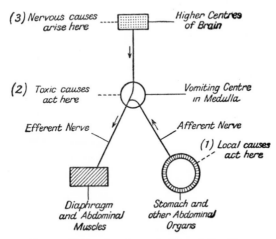

FIG. 2—Illustrating the mechanism of Vomiting.

In order to appreciate their mode of action it is necessary to recall the physiological mechanism of vomiting.

There is a special vomiting centre in the medulla oblongata to which pass afferent (sensory) nerves from the stomach and other abdominal viscera. From the centre the efferent (motor) nerves are distributed to the muscle of the stomach, the diaphragm and the muscles of the abdominal wall, all of which take part in the muscular effort associated with vomiting. There is, therefore, a reflex arc through the vomiting centre from the sensory organ (the mucous membrane of the stomach) to the motor organs just mentioned. The centre is also connected to the higher centres of the brain, including those of sight and smell.

Vomiting may be produced:

(1) by stimuli which arise in the stomach or other parts of the alimentary system and pass to the vomiting centre;

(2) the centre itself may be affected by drugs or toxins;

(3) the centre may receive stimuli from the higher centres, such as those produced by revolting sights and smells.

## Sedatives and anti-emetics

These are drugs which either tend to diminish the movements of the stomach or else to depress the vomiting centre. They include:

(a) Drugs of the anti-histamine type viz:
   Promethazine ('Avomine')
   Cyclizine ('Marzine')  } 25-50 mg.
   Dimenhydrinate ('Dramamine')

(b) Drugs of the promazine group:
   Promazine ('Sparine')  } 25-50 mg.
   Chlorpromazine ('Largactil') } as anti-emetics.
   Perphenazine ('Fentazin'), 2-4 mg.

The first group are particularly useful in the prevention and treatment of travel sickness and both groups in vomiting of pregnancy and that due to other causes. Some of these drugs may also be given by intramuscular injection.

(c) Simple drugs which may be used include 'Chlorodyne' (*Tinctura chloroformi et morphinæ* 0·6 ml. (5-10 minims), chlorbutol ('chloretone') 1·2 gram (5-20 gr.), atropine and belladonna, and also barbiturates.

Kaolin and morphine mixture may be used, especially if diarrhœa is present.

## Stomachics, including bitters

These are given with a view to stimulating the appetite and the secretion of gastric juice, thereby improving digestion and aiding the general nutrition, especially during convalescence. They include gentian, nux vomica and quinine.

## Antacids

These drugs are given in order to neutralize hydrochloric acid in cases of gastric and duodenal ulcer or to neutralize its excess in hyperchlorhydria and in the symptomatic treatment of heartburn. The most important are:

| | |
|---|---|
| Magnesia (magnesium oxide). | Aluminium hydroxide. |
| Magnesium carbonate. | Aluminium glycinate ('Prodexin'). |
| Magnesium phosphate. | Bismuth carbonate. |
| Magnesium trisilicate. | Sodium bicarbonate. |

Aluminium hydroxide (sometimes used in the form of 'Aludrox') may also be given as a colloidal solution by the continuous drip method through a nasal catheter.

Sodium bicarbonate in the presence of hydrochloric acid liberates carbon dioxide and later stimulates the further secretion of hydrochloric acid, so is unsuitable for use alone as an antacid.

A number of the above substances may be mixed together to form special antacid powders, e.g.

(i) Magnesium trisilicate        (ii) Magnesium carbonate
    Magnesium carbonate               Calcium carbonate
    Sodium bicarbonate                Bismuth carbonate
    Calcium carbonate

The doses of the majority of these powders and drugs varies between 2 and 4 grams (30-60 grains).

It must be remembered that some of them tend to have a laxative action which, in certain individuals, is sufficient to cause considerable discomfort. Magnesium trisilicate is free from this defect. (N.B.—Mist. Mag. Trisil., N.F., contains only 600 mg. (10 grains) of magnesium trisilicate in each 15 ml. ($\frac{1}{2}$ oz.) dose.) Others given in large doses may produce the condition of alkalosis.

Special compressed tablets consisting of various alkalis which are allowed to dissolve slowly in the mouth between the cheek and lower jaw at the rate of two an hour are an effective means of neutralizing the acid of the gastric juice. (e.g. 'Nulacin', 'Gelusil', 'Prodexin.')

Atropine and belladonna, 'Probanthine' (propantheline) and 'Antrenyl' also diminish the secretion of hydrochloric acid, not by a direct chemical action but by a sedative action on the nervous mechanism of its secretion. 'Nacton' is also useful.

### Substitutes

(a) Pepsin may be given as an aid to digestion when it is considered that the secretion of pepsin may be defective, e.g. *Mistura bismuthi cum pepsino*.

(b) Dilute hydrochloric acid (*Acidum hydrochloricum dilutum*, 4 ml., 5 to 60 minims) may be given in water or orange juice with meals in cases of achlorhydria or hypochlorhydria and is useful in checking the diarrhœa which sometimes accompanies these conditions.

### Drugs used in radiography of the stomach

A suspension of barium sulphate, which is opaque to X-rays, is generally employed. It is swallowed as a "barium meal", which can be followed by radiography in its course through the œsophagus, stomach, small and large intestines. In addition to showing the outline of the organs this also gives information about their rate of emptying. A "barium enema" is given for examination of the rectum and colon.

## Other drugs used for their action on the stomach

### Atropine Methonitrate ('Eumydrin')

As its chemical name implies, this drug is a salt of atropine in composition and has similar actions. It is of special value, however, in being less toxic and more effective in the medical treatment of congenital hypertrophic pyloric stenosis than atropine. By its action it helps to relax the hypertrophied pyloric sphincter and to allow the passage of the stomach contents into the duodenum. It is of value also in relieving the spasms of whooping cough. It may be given in the following ways:

(i) 0·12 to 2 ml. of 0·6 per cent alcoholic solution given on the tongue before each feed. This solution is very potent and must be used with great care. The container must be kept tightly closed to prevent evaporation and must not be confused with atropine methonitrate eye drops. It is unsuitable for out-patients.

(ii) 1 to 4 ml. of a 1 in 10,000 aqueous solution, half an hour before each feed. This is continued for some weeks. The solution must be made up fresh every three days.

(iii) Lamellæ or gelatin discs containing $\frac{1}{750}$ grain placed under the tongue 15 minutes before each feed.

### *The test meal*

**Charcoal** biscuits are sometimes given on the night before the test. A residue of charcoal in the resting juice the following morning indicates that the stomach is not emptying properly, i.e. pyloric stenosis.

**Histamine.** A subcutaneous injection of 0·5 to 1 ml. of a 1 in 1000 solution (0·5 mg.) is given in certain cases to prove the presence of achylia gastrica, in which there is the complete absence of hydrochloric acid from the gastric juice. Hydrochloric acid may be absent from the juice (achlorhydria), although the stomach is still capable of secreting it. In such instances, histamine will stimulate the glands of the gastric mucous membrane to secrete hydrochloric acid and thereby prove that the case is not one of true achylia gastrica.

*The alcohol test meal.* Instead of the usual gruel test meal, 50 ml. of 7 per cent alcohol may be given.

## DRUGS ACTING ON THE INTESTINES

1. Those promoting evacuation. (The aperients, enemata and suppositories.)
2. Those which lessen movements and spasm. (Sedatives.)
3. Intestinal antiseptics.
4. Those destroying worm parasites—anthelmintics.

### The aperients

An aperient is a drug employed in medicine to assist the bowel to evacuate its contents and, in the majority of instances, it does so on account of its power of stimulating peristalsis and the movements of the bowel.

It will be recalled that the onward passage of the intestinal contents is due to two main factors: (1) Peristalsis. (2) The operation of the important gastro-colic reflex. When food is taken into the stomach this causes a reflex relaxation of the ileo-cæcal valve by which the contents of the lower ileum rapidly enter the cæcum and, as a result, the contents of the colon are passed on into the rectum. The distension of the rectum thus produced give rise to the natural desire to defæcate.

Aperients are sometimes classified according to the intensity of their action thus:

*1. Laxatives.* These are relatively mild and result in the hastening of peristaltic action without altering the appearance or consistency of the stools. Simple lubricants such as liquid paraffin may also be included in this group.

*2. Mild purgatives.* These are stronger in action, producing looser and, sometimes, repeated stools.

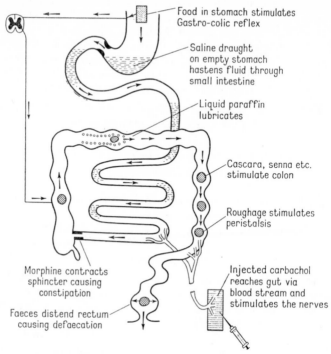

Food in stomach stimulates Gastro-colic reflex

Saline draught on empty stomach hastens fluid through small intestine

Liquid paraffin lubricates

Cascara, senna etc. stimulate colon

Roughage stimulates peristalsis

Injected carbachol reaches gut via blood stream and stimulates the nerves

Morphine contracts sphincter causing constipation

Faeces distend rectum causing defaecation

FIG. 3—Diagram illustrating the action of some aperients.

**3. Drastic purgatives.** These are violent in action, often accompanied by pain and colic, and resulting in frequent and watery stools comparable with those of acute enteritis.

This classification is to some extent an artificial one because, in a number of instances, the effect produced is dependent upon the dose of the drug administered and, in excessive doses, some of the milder laxatives may act as drastic purgatives. However, from a practical point of view it is useful if the recognized doses of the various drugs are adhered to. The term aperient has here been used to cover all the groups.

### Modes of action

Aperients act in various ways.

(i) The principal natural stimulus to peristalsis is the presence of fæcal material stretching the muscle of the intestinal wall. Peristalsis is, therefore, more active if the amount of fæcal residue is increased. In addition to taking vegetable and cellulose material in the diet to produce "roughage", the bulk of the fæces may be increased by non-absorbable substances, such as agar, which swell as they take up water present in the gut.

(ii) Certain aperients, particularly those of the saline group, e.g. Epsom salts (magnesium sulphate), act mainly as hypertonic solutions which withdraw fluid via the mucous membrane of the gut. This fluid increases the bulk of the stool. At the same time the increased bulk of the stool causes more rapid peristalsis and, therefore, there is less time for the normal absorption of fluid from the lower bowel.

(iii) Others act by stimulating the nervous mechanism of peristalsis.

(iv) The drastic purgatives produce a definite inflammatory reaction in the mucous membrane of the intestine which results not only in stimulation of peristalsis but also in the outpouring of an inflammatory exudate. This also increases the relative bulk of the intestinal contents and, in addition, the hurried passage of the contents along the gut does not permit time for the normal absorption of fluid mentioned above. Frequent, copious and watery stools are, therefore, obtained.

In some instances the action of the drugs is more marked on the small intestine, in others it is on the large intestine. The main result, however, is to produce a rapid distension of the rectum with the contents of the gut above, which is very similar to the effect of an enema distending the rectum when given from below.

SUMMARY. The effects of aperients are:

1. To increase the active movements of the intestine, i.e. to stimulate peristalsis and to hurry the passage of the intestinal contents.

2. By mild irritation of the intestinal mucous membrane to increase either slightly or greatly the amount of fluid exudate from the mucosa.

3. To hasten the progress of the intestinal contents so that the normal absorption of water by the colon is partially prevented.

4. To produce rapid distension of the rectum and the associated desire to defæcate.

Since the majority of aperients cause mild irritation of the mucous membrane of the gut it should be clear that their habitual use is undesirable. Their constant employment may cause the natural functions of the intestine to become sluggish so that a vicious circle is set up. It is a common experience that individuals who always employ aperients need to take constantly increasing doses of more powerful drugs.

In comparison with acute constipation associated with some temporary disorder or disease, chronic constipation (dyschezia) is, in most instances, due to faulty habits and failure to respond to the natural call to defæcate which occurs when the rectum becomes distended. The ideal treatment of chronic constipation is therefore not the regular administration of aperients but the gradual re-education of the bowel. This can generally be obtained by (a) regular attempts at evacuation assisted by providing an adequate bulk of the fæces in the form of roughage, and (b) simple enemata from the use of which the patient is gradually weaned. (c) Glycerin or bisacodyl ('Dulcolax') suppositories are useful in some cases. Aperients may be of some value at the commencement of the course but should be dropped as soon as possible.

## 1. Laxatives

### Roughage

As already mentioned, the natural stimulus of peristalsis is an adequate bulk of the fæces in the form of food residue consisting mainly of undigested cellulose. Wholemeal bread, vegetables, and fruits, especially figs and prunes, are all of value for this purpose.

### Agar

This is prepared from various sea-weeds. It is not altered by digestion but has the power of absorbing water. In so doing it expands considerably in bulk and, by increasing the

volume of the fæces, it promotes peristalsis. Agar is sometimes mixed with liquid paraffin to form an emulsion. 'Nor-
macol', 'Isogel', 'Metamucil' and various plant mucilages have
a similar action.

## Liquid paraffin

This is a bland mineral oil which passes through the
intestinal tract unchanged by the processes of digestion. It
has no action on the mucous membrane of the gut, but acts
as a simple lubricant, softening the fæces and aiding their
passage through the bowel and rectum. There is no advantage
in giving excessive doses and, when it appears to "run through"
the patient, the dose should be appropriately reduced. The
usual dose is 30 ml. ($\frac{1}{2}$ to 1 ounce) at night, or possibly night
and morning. Liquid paraffin emulsion is a useful preparation.

Its prolonged use may possibly lead to vitamin deficiency
by interfering with their absorption.

Magnesium hydroxide and syrup of figs (*Syrupus ficorum*,
8 ml., 30 to 120 minims) are also laxatives especially useful for
children.

### 2. *Mild purgatives*

In smaller doses the following drugs will acts as laxatives,
but in full doses they are mild purgatives.

### (a) *Saline aperients*

The saline aperients act fairly quickly and are best given
in warm water on an empty stomach before breakfast.

Sodium sulphate (*Sodii sulphas*, Glauber's salt), 16 grams
(30 to 240 grains).

Magnesium sulphate (*Magnesii sulphas*, Epsom salts), 16
grams (30 to 240 grains).

White mixture (*Mistura magnesii sulphatis alba*, B.P.C.), contains magnesium sulphate (4 grams, 60 grains) and light
magnesium carbonate (0·6 gram, 10 grains, to 15 ml., $\frac{1}{2}$
ounce) of peppermint water.

Seidlitz powder (*Pulvis effervescens compositus*, B.P.C.) consists of
sodium potassium tartrate and sodium bicarbonate in the blue packet
and tartaric acid in the white packet. The contents of the blue packet
are dissolved in half a pint of cold or warm water; those of the white
packet are then added and the draught taken while effervescing.

## (b) *Drugs of the senna, cascara, rhubarb and aloes group*

These are all mild purgatives of vegetable origin which do not produce inflammation of the intestine like the drugs of the drastic purgative group. As a rule they take 10 to 18 hours to produce an effect. Owing to some absorption from the bowel and subsequent excretion in the urine, rhubarb and senna tend to impart to the latter a yellow-brown colour.

### Senna

This may be prepared from the leaflets or pods of the plant. It tends to produce more griping than other members of the group and its main action is on the colon. Important preparations include:

Senna pods, 2 gm. (10 to 30 grains) or 4 to 12 pods.

Syrup of senna (*Syrupus sennæ*), 8 ml. (30 to 120 minims).

Black draught (*Mistura sennæ composita*), 30 ml. (1 to 2 ounces).

'Senokot' is a most useful proprietary preparation.

### Cascara sagrada

This is a bark from which the following important preparations are made:

Cascara sagrada elixir (*Elixir cascaræ sagradæ*, B.P.), 4 ml. (30 to 60 minims).

Compound cascara mixture (*Mistura cascaræ et belladonnæ*, B.P.C.), 15 ml. (½ ounce).

Compound cascara sagrada tablet (*Tabella cascaræ sagradæ composita*, B.P.C.), 1 or 2 tablets.

### Rhubarb (*Rheum*)

This is a rhizome from which the following preparations are made:
Compound rhubarb pill (*Pilula rhei composita*, B.P.).

It is also made up as rhubarb and soda mixture (*Mistura rhei composita*, B.P.C.), 15 ml. (½ ounce).

### Aloes

This is a dried juice obtained from the leaves of aloes plants. Preparations include:

Aloes and nux vomica tablet (*Tab. aloes et nucis vomicæ*, B.P.C.), 1 tablet.

## Phenolphthalein

This is a synthetic drug similar in action to the vegetable drugs mentioned above. It is given in doses of up to 300 mg. (1 to 5 grains). Phenaloin pill consists of a mixture of aloes, phenolphthalein, strychnine and belladonna (1 to 3 pills). Belladonna is added to prevent griping.

*Bisacodyl* ('Dulcolax'), one or two tablets of 5 mg., is a useful and popular aperient also employed as a suppository.

## Castor oil (*Oleum ricini*)

Applied to the surface of the body, castor oil is a bland substance having an emollient action. It is also used to allay irritation in the eye and, mixed with zinc oxide, as an application to the skin.

In the intestines, however, it is altered in composition by the pancreatic enzymes and substances are produced which have a mildly irritating effect on the intestine, thereby giving the drug its aperient action. It may be given in capsules, as an emulsion, or mixture and various devices have been mentioned (page 25) for disguising its taste.

After its aperient action has passed off it tends to have a slightly constipating effect, hence its use in diarrhœa due to poisonous or unsuitable food, when it may be given with a view to emptying the intestine rapidly (2-6 hours) and then checking the condition by its constipating action. It is sometimes given after abdominal operations. Dose up to 30 ml. (1 fluid ounce).

### *3. Drastic purgatives or cathartics*

These drugs are now rarely employed. They include:

Calomel.    Jalap.    Colocynth.

## Calomel (*Hydrargyri subchloridum*, Mercurous chloride)

Calomel must not be confused with corrosive sublimate (*Hydrargyri perchloridum*, Mercuric chloride, page 40). It is usually given at night and followed by a saline draught before breakfast to prevent the absorption of any mercury. Two methods of administration are employed: (i) repeated small doses, e.g. 16 mg. (¼ grain) every hour until the bowels are open; (ii) a single dose of 0·3 gram (1 to 5 grains). A moderate dose, for example, 0·2 gram (3 grains), is often less painful than a smaller dose of 60 mg. (1 grain). There is a danger of producing collapse in some patients after full doses.

## Colocynth

This is given as:

Colocynth and hyoscyamus pill (*Pilula colocynthidis et hyoscyami*, B.P.), dose, 1 or 2 pills.

The hyoscyamus is added to lessen the griping effect of colocynth.

### Drugs given by hypodermic injection

Certain drugs, having an action on the neuro-muscular mechanism of the bowel whereby they increase the tone of the intestinal muscle and stimulate its movements, may be given by hypodermic injection. They are especially useful in post-operative abdominal distension. They include:

Pituitary, posterior lobe injection ('Pituitrin') (0·5 ml.).

Neostigmine injection (0·5 to 2 mg.).

Carbachol ('Doryl', 'Moryl') (0·5 mg., $\frac{1}{240}$ to $\frac{1}{120}$ grain). The last named are most used and are also employed to stimulate the tone of the stomach muscle in acute dilatation of the stomach.

### Enemata

An enema consists of the injection of fluid into the rectum. Enemas may be given in order to empty the lower bowel, or for other purposes.

The main points to be remembered in the administration of rectal injections are:

(i) Collect all the required apparatus on a tray and cover with a towel before approaching the patient.

(ii) Whenever possible, place the patient in the lateral position. Enemata may be given with the patient on his back or in the knee-elbow position if necessary.

(iii) Do not insert the nozzle of a Higginson's syringe directly into the anus but attach a soft rubber catheter, which may be lubricated with a little 'Vaseline' spread on lint, and inserted into the rectum for two inches. The tube and funnel method is, however, usually employed.

(iv) Fluids should be injected at a temperature of 98-100°F., (37°C.) unless otherwise prescribed.

(v) After the removal of the catheter the patient should be lifted on to the bed-pan.

TYPES OF ENEMATA.

1. Those to be returned ⎰ warm water.   arachis oil.
          evacuant ⎨ soap.        glycerin.
               ⎰ turpentine.   calcium chloride.

2. Those to be retained.
    (a) sedative    . starch and opium.
    (b) anæsthetic  . bromethol ('Avertin').

The following are the common types of enemata given:

1. Warm water enema.

2. Soap enema (1 ounce of soft soap to 20 ounces of warm water).

3. Turpentine enema (15 ml., 1 ounce, of oil of turpentine is added to the soap enema; or 15 ml., 1 ounce, of oil of turpentine to 360 ml., 12 ounces, of thin starch mucilage). This is especially useful in aiding the removal of flatus and after abdominal operations.

Turpentine has a deleterious effect on rubber and this enema is preferably given with a tube and funnel. If a Higginson's syringe is used it should be cleaned immediately.

4. Calcium chloride, 120 ml. (4 fl. oz.) of 5% solution causes an immediate evacuation and is useful in the management of elderly incontinent patients.

5. Arachis oil enema. Up to 300 ml. (5 to 10 ounces) of arachis oil are warmed in a water bath to 98°F., and run into the rectum by a tube and funnel. It should be retained from $\frac{1}{2}$ to 1 hour and may be followed in 4 hours by a soap enema if necessary. Olive oil may be used but is more expensive.

6. Glycerin enema. 8 ml. (60 to 120 minims) of glycerin are introduced by means of a catheter attached to a suitable syringe. A glycerin suppository has a similar effect.

7. Sedative enema. This is sometimes given to check excessive diarrhœa. The one employed is the starch and opium enema. For an adult 140 ml. (5 ounces) of thin starch mucilage containing 2·5 ml. (40 minims) of tincture of opium

are introduced at a temperature of 100°F. by the tube-and-funnel method.

(To make thin starch mucilage, take a tablespoonful of starch powder and mix with a little cold water, make this up to 10 ounces with boiling water and allow to cool.)

**Enema rash.** Occasionally a patchy erythematous rash develops about 12 hours after an enema has been given. It usually appears on the face, buttocks and knees and may last for 24 hours. It is sometimes mistaken for scarlet fever or measles, but there is no pyrexia, it is not irritating and, as a rule, requires no treatment. Calamine lotion may be applied if desired.

### Suppositories

Glycerine and bisacodyl ('Dulcolax') are useful evacuant suppositories which are often used instead of enemata.

### Intestinal sedatives

Intestinal sedatives have an opposite action to aperients, for they lessen peristaltic movement and diminish spasm. They are used in enteritis to check diarrhœa, to soothe the mucous membrane and to relieve colic. They may be classified thus:

### (a) Soothing agents

Kaolin, bismuth salts and magnesium trisilicate are examples of drugs which help to protect the mucous membrane by their soothing action.

Kaolin and charcoal also adsorb intestinal gases and prevent over-distension of the bowel, thus diminishing its movement and the colicky pains which are caused by the distension.

### (b) Drugs acting on nervous mechanism

Atropine and belladonna, and morphine and opium all act on the nervous mechanism. Atropine helps to relax spasm, while morphine has a general depressing effect on the muscular movements and tends to produce constipation.

Proprietary preparations which have an antispasmodic

action on the alimentary tract include propantheline ('Prob-anthine'), 'Antrenyl', 'Merbentyl', 'Wyovin'.

Among the most useful remedies for diarrhœa are mixtures containing kaolin or bismuth salts and a small dose of mor-phine, e.g. *Mistura Kaolini et Morphinæ*; and Chlorodyne (p. 156). Codein phosphate (60 mg., 1 gr.) may be of value. For infective cases sulphonamides are often employed.

Diarrhœa associated with achlorhydria sometimes responds to the administration of hydrochloric acid (page 67).

## Antiparasitic Drugs

(a) Intestinal antiseptics.
(b) Anthelmintics.

### 1. Intestinal antiseptics

Under normal circumstances the presence of hydrochloric acid in the stomach renders its contents sterile, and in health this freedom from living organisms is maintained throughout the upper part of the small intestine. From the lower end of the ileum, however, the number of bacteria present increases and they are very numerous in the colon. Here they normally play an important part in the digestive processes by helping to break down cellulose, which is unaffected by the digestive juices in the stomach and small intestine.

Sometimes bacteria pass through the hydrochloric acid barrier and cause inflammation of the intestine (enteritis) or special conditions such as typhoid fever, bacillary dysentery and food poisoning. The bacteria which may be found in the intestines may, therefore, be classified as (a) pathogenic, or those responsible for disease of the intestines and (b) non-pathogenic, that is those organisms which are normally present in the intestines but cause no disease when they are confined to the bowel. They may, however, be harmful if they reach the peritoneum or other tissues. Included in this group are the organisms which assist in the digestion of cellulose in the colon. In certain circumstances these organisms may cause excessive putrefaction of the bowel contents or excessive fer-mentation, with the production of gas, some of which may be absorbed by kaolin or charcoal.

The usual method of treatment employed in a case of food poisoning or severe diarrhœa is:

(i) In some cases to get rid of the infected material as soon as possible by an aperient, e.g. castor oil, supplemented if necessary by lavage of the colon with normal saline.

(ii) To allay the irritation of the mucous membrane by a mixture containing kaolin and morphine.

(iii) To relieve pain and spasm, if necessary, with morphine and atropine.

(iv) To absorb gas and intestinal toxins by charcoal or kaolin.

(v) To replace the fluid lost from the body by diarrhœa by giving fluids orally, subcutaneously or intravenously.

(vi) To avoid further irritation of the bowel by giving a light and easily digested diet commencing with milk, gruel and arrowroot.

(vii) To give one of the sulphonamides or antibiotics by mouth if a definite organism is found to be responsible for the condition.

Sulphonamides, including the insoluble ones which are not absorbed from the bowel such as sulphaguanidine, 'Sulphasuxidine' and 'Sulphathalidine', affect the growth of intestinal bacteria. A popular preparation is 'Guanimycin' (a mixture of Sulphagnanidine and Streptomycin). Tetracycline, chloramphenicol, etc., when given by mouth destroy many bacteria in the intestines (page 236). If given for more than a few days, however, not only do they permit the overgrowth of many bacteria which are insensitive to them but they may also seriously affect the absorption of certain vitamins, particularly these of the vitamin B complex. Preparations of vitamin B must, therefore, be given at the same time if their administration is prolonged. Erythromycin is particularly valuable in cases of enteritis caused by staphylococci.

## Treatment of special bowel infections
### Dysentery

There are two types of dysentery:

(a) Amœbic dysentery caused by a single-celled organism known as the *Entamœba histolytica*. In addition to general symptomatic treatment, emetine (60 mg., 1 grain, daily for 12 doses) is given by subcutaneous or intramuscular injection. Emetine is extracted from ipecacuanha.

(b) Bacillary dysentery. Sulphaguanidine, 'Sulphasuxidine' and sulphadiazine are used. Tetracycline is also effective.

## 2. Anthelmintics

The intestinal canal may become the home of various parasitic worms. The ova or eggs of the parasites usually enter the human being (the host) in contaminated food or water. They reach the intestine, where they mature into the fully grown worm.

Drugs used in the treatment of worms are called **anthelmintics.** Those which actually kill the worm are sometimes referred to as **vermicides** while those which merely cause its expulsion from the body are called **vermifuges.**

The following are the most important varieties of worm found:

| | |
|---|---|
| Thread worms. | Tape worms. |
| Round worms. | Hook worms. |

### Thread Worms (*Oxyuris vermicularis*).

These are common in children and inhabit the large intestine. Their successful eradication depends entirely upon the prevention of reinfection. Their presence is often associated with itching of the anus, for which benzocaine ointment may be applied. Other members of the household should also be checked for the presence of worms or ova.

*Treatment:*

(i) **Gentian violet** (*Viola crystallina*) given in enteric-coated capsules is one of the most effective remedies. The adult dose is 60 mg. (1 grain), t.d.s. with meals; for children up to 10 mg. ($\frac{1}{6}$ grain) for each year of age. Two courses each lasting eight days with an interval of a week are given.

(ii) **Piperazine** is also used, e.g. 'Antipar', 'Helmezine', 'Entacyl'.

(iii) **Diphenan** ('Butolan', 'Oxylan') have been used.

Treatment may be commenced by giving one or two enemas, using either saline (1 or 2 tablespoonful of salt to one pint) or infusion of quassia (6 to 10 ounces) which will help to get rid of some of the worms and, if given at night, may relieve itching of the anus but will not cure the condition.

### Round Worms (*Ascaris lumbricoides*)

These resemble the earth worm in appearance and, in addition to entering the intestine, may occasionally wander into the stomach from which they may be vomited, or into the bile ducts when they produce jaundice.

*Treatment.* The following drugs are used:

(i) **Piperazine** is the safest drug to use. A single dose of 4 grams may be given to an adult. For children the dose is calculated according to the age and weight. No purgative is necessary unless constipation is present.

(ii) **Santonin** (10 mg., $\frac{1}{6}$ grain, for each year up to 0·2 gram, 3 grains). It is generally given on two or three nights, and followed by castor oil, calomel or saline aperient in the morning. It does not actually kill the worm, which is expelled alive, and is therefore a vermifuge. It turns the urine bright yellow if acid, and purple if alkaline and the patient may complain of yellow vision (xanthopsia).

### Tape Worms (*Tænia solium, Tænia saginata*)

The effective treatment of tape worms requires careful adherence to a strict routine. The drugs most commonly employed are male fern (*Filix mas*) and mepacrine.

(i) **Male Fern.** In order that the anthelmintic drug may come into full contact with the worm, it is necessary for the stomach and intestines to be as empty as possible. The patient is, therefore, starved for 2 days, fluids only being given. Saline aperients are taken each morning. On the third morning, 6 ml. (45 to 90 minims) of the liquid extract of male fern (*Extractum filicis*) is given and followed 2 hours later by 120 grains (8 grams) of magnesium sulphate. If the bowels are not opened within an hour or so, a soap and water enema is administered.

The motions should be collected in warm water and a

search made for the head of the worm. If it is not found the treatment should be repeated in 10 days.

Under no circumstances should castor oil be given after *Filix mas*, as a combination of these drugs produces very dangerous toxic symptoms.

(ii) **Mepacrine hydrochloride.** This drug which is used in the treatment of malaria is also effective against tape worms. 100 mg. are given every five minutes for ten doses (total 1 gram). Its action is less certain than that of male fern.

### Hook Worms *(Ancylostoma)*

The ova of these worms may be found in the fæces of patients from tropical countries. The larvæ bore their way through the skin and reach the duodenum via the blood vessels, lungs and trachea, causing anæmia and eosinophilia. 'Alcopar', 5 gram in 15 ml. ($\frac{1}{2}$ oz.) of water three times a day before meals for one day, repeated in one week is used in treatment.

Other anthelmintics include (adult doses):
Carbon tetrachloride (up to 3 ml.) for hook worm.
Tetrachlorethylene, up to 6 ml. for round and hook worm.

## DRUGS ACTING ON THE LIVER AND BILIARY APPARATUS

There are few drugs which can be used to alter the functions of the liver or to increase the formation of bile, but certain substances hasten the evacuation of bile from the gall-bladder into the duodenum. They are called *cholagogues* and include:

Sodium salicylate (2 grams, 10 to 30 grains), sodium sulphate (16 grams, 120 to 240 grains) and magnesium sulphate (30 to 240 grains).

Sulphonamides and antibiotics are the most effective biliary antiseptics.

The injection of adrenaline (1 in 1000) causes the liver to convert the glycogen stored in it into glucose, which passes into the blood. This fact is sometimes made use of in the treatment of hypoglycæmia due to overdosage of insulin.

A fatty meal or the administration of olive oil into the stomach or duodenum causes the gall-bladder to empty its contents into the duodenum.

Glucose is said to have a "protective" action on the liver and helps to diminish the damage done to the organ in various toxic states. Calcium gluconate is also given for the same purpose but it is difficult to explain their mode of action, if any.

### Cholecystography

Iodophthalein, or one of the proprietary preparations such as Telepaque, Pheniodol or Opacol, when given by mouth, are absorbed in the alimentary tract and excreted by the liver into the bile. For a time they are stored and concentrated in the gall-bladder. These substances are opaque to X-rays and a radiogram can therefore be obtained showing the outline of the gall-bladder, provided it is functioning normally.

*Technique.* On the day before the examination is carried out, the amount of fat in the diet is reduced to a minimum. The patient has a light supper containing no fat at 7 p.m. At 10 p.m. the dye dissolved in water is given, followed by further drinks of water. The patient is instructed to lie on his right side. X-ray pictures are taken next day, 14, 18 and 19 hours after the dye has been given (i.e. 12 noon, 4 p.m., 5 p.m.). During this period no food is allowed, but water may be drunk. The first meal is given one hour (i.e. after the 4 p.m. radiogram) before the last X-ray. This consists of a fatty meal which should contain bread, butter, bacon and a cup of tea. Alternatively a fat emulsion containing nut oil ('Prosparol'), dose: 120 ml., 4 fl. oz., may be used.

'Biligrafin' may be given intravenously.

### Test of liver function. Lævulose tolerance test.

In a normal individual there is little or no rise in the blood-sugar taken one hour after 50 grams of lævulose have been given by mouth in 100 ml. of water. If the functions of the liver are defective, the blood-sugar shows a rise from the normal of 120 mg. per 100 ml. to 140 to 190 mg. per 100 ml.

Other liver function tests include the Van den Burgh reaction which involves the estimation of the serum bilirubin, estimation of the blood proteins (albumin and globulin) and various chemical tests carried out on the blood.

# CHAPTER 7

# THE ACTION OF DRUGS ON THE HEART AND CIRCULATION

In order to understand the action of drugs on the heart and circulatory system it is necessary to review certain aspects of their physiology.

1. The heart-muscle acts as a pump which supplies the motive force, driving the blood under pressure through the arterial system to all the organs and tissues of the body where it is distributed in the capillaries. The veins are the "return" channels of the circulatory system.

The volume of blood passing through the heart each minute is called the cardiac output. In health cardiac output varies according to the immediate needs of the body, being increased on exercise by an increase in the rate and force with which the heart beats.

In cardiac failure, when the myocardium can no longer supply sufficient force, the cardiac output is reduced. This leads to:

(i) Inadequate blood supply to the organs and tissues.

(ii) Diminished activity of the kidneys causing salt and water retention and œdema.

(iii) Venous congestion.

2. In order to act efficiently the muscle must be adequately nourished. In particular, it requires oxygen and glucose to satisfy its metabolic needs. These reach it in the blood supplied to it through the coronary arteries. Diminution in the size of the lumen of the coronary arteries, either temporarily as a result of spasm or permanently owing to disease of their walls, will result in defective nutrition of the heart-muscle, with either temporary or permanent effects on its efficiency.

3. The pressure of blood within the arteries is dependent on (i) the force of the heart beat, i.e. the strength of the muscular contraction, (ii) the calibre of the arteries, (iii) the

elasticity of the arteries, i.e. if the arteries are narrowed and inelastic the blood pressure is raised.

4. The rhythm of the heart and the orderly sequence with which the various chambers contract is dependent on specialized neuro-muscular tissue in the heart.

The impulse for each cardiac contraction commences at the sino-atrial node (the pacemaker of the heart) near the entrance of the superior vena cava into the right atrium. It spreads over the muscle of both atria and reaches the atrio-ventricular node, from which it passes down the atrio-ventricular bundle of His. Towards the lower end of the inter-ventricular septum, the bundle of His divides into right and left branches and distributes the impulse to contract to the right and left ventricles respectively.

The bundle of His can only pass a certain number of impulses per minute, that is to say, a definite period must elapse after one impulse has passed before the bundle is able to transmit the next. This period of rest during which no impulse can pass is called the refractory period.

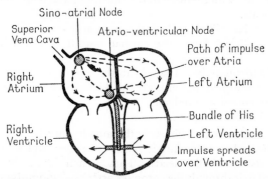

Fig. 4.—Illustrating the spread of the impulse for contraction from the sino-atrial node over the auricles to reach the atrio-ventricular node, whence it passes down the bundle of His and is distributed to the ventricles.

5. The constant rate of the heart is maintained because the sino-atrial node is under the influence of two sets of nervous impulses which normally are equally balanced.

Para-sympathetic nerve-fibres reaching the heart in the

vagus (Xth cranial) nerve carry impulses which tend to slow its rate (inhibitors).

Sympathetic fibres from the cardiac plexus tend to increase its rate (accelerators).

Therefore, drugs which tend to paralyse or depress the para-sympathetic or vagus will permit over-action of the sympathetic and the rate of the heart will be increased. Those which stimulate the vagus (para-sympathetic) will slow the rate.

Conversely, stimulation of the sympathetic fibres will also increase the heart-rate, while their depression will slow the rate by permitting over-action of the vagus.

As an example, adrenaline, which stimulates the sympathetic, will increase the rate of the heart if given by injection or if its secretion by the suprarenal glands is naturally increased as it is in states of fear or violent emotion.

## DRUGS ACTING ON THE HEART

The most important drugs acting on the heart itself are those of the digitalis group, and the condition on which they have the most beneficial and dramatic effect is atrial (auricular) *fibrillation*.

In atrial fibrillation, the atrial muscle loses its power of contracting as a whole, and instead of one impulse commencing at the sino-atrial node spreading in an orderly fashion over the atrial muscle to reach the atrio-ventricular node at the rate of approximately 72 per minute, a series of irregular contractions occur which are scattered over the atria. Each of these small contractions produces an impulse which passes to the atrio-ventricular node. In atrial fibrillation, therefore, this node is bombarded with impulses at the rate of about 400 per minute.

Owing to the refractory period, however, the bundle of His can only transmit a certain number of these irregular impulses. The ventricle therefore contracts at irregular intervals at a rapid rate (often up to 130 beats per minute).

Since the contractions of the ventricle occur at irregular and rapid intervals, it follows that it can never be filled completely nor will it contain the same amount of blood for each beat. Therefore the output per beat is small and variable in quantity. This means that the pulse will also be irregular both in rhythm and volume. Some of the heart beats will be so small that the pulse-wave produced will be imperceptible at the wrist. Therefore the rate of the pulse counted at the wrist will not be a true indication of the rate of the ventricles. Hence the importance of taking and recording both the pulse-rate and the rate at the apex in cases of atrial fibrillation.

### The digitalis group

Drugs of the digitalis group act: (i) on the bundle of His in auricular fibrillation. Their action is a depressing one, that is, they lower its power of conducting impulses. In other words, they increase the refractory period. By this means, the bundle of His allows fewer of the irregular impulses bombarding the atrio-ventricular node to pass and, by adjusting the dose of the drug, this number can be reduced to 70 or 80 per minute or even lower.

In this way the ventricular rate is slowed. Slowing of the ventricle means better filling of the ventricle and an increased output per beat. Consequently, the efficiency of the heart as a pump is increased and the general circulation is improved. (ii) Digitalis acts directly on the myocardium and increases the force of systotic contraction. It thereby increases cardiac output and reduces venous congestion and the raised venous pressure in congestive heart failure.

The improvement in the circulation has other beneficial effects:

(1) The circulation in the coronary arteries is increased and the nutrition of the heart is improved.

(2) The circulation in the kidneys is improved and the output of urine is increased, a factor important in the reduction of cardiac œdema. This explains the diuretic action of digitalis in heart disease.

(3) Œdema is also diminished, by reason of the improved circulation in the more distant and dependent parts of the body.

SUMMARY

The action of the digitalis group of drugs may be summarized:

(i) Digitalis is of special value in atrial (auricular) fibrillation.

(ii) It acts by depressing the bundle of His and increasing its refractory period.

(iii) Thereby it slows ventricular rate, increases the output per beat and improves the circulation.

(iv) Digitalis also has a general tonic effect on the heart-muscle, increasing the force of ventricular contraction and the cardiac output. It is, therefore, of value in other cases of cardiac weakness. Its most dramatic effect, however, is in atrial fibrillation.

(v) Improvement in the circulation has a beneficial effect on various symptoms, e.g. the urinary output is increased; œdema is diminished.

(vi) It has some action on the vagus nerve and sino-atrial node which also contributes to the slowing of the cardiac rate.

(vii) In therapeutic doses digitalis has little action on the normal heart.

## Digitalis

Digitalis is obtained from the foxglove (*Digitalis purpurea*) and was first used in the treatment of heart disease by Withering in 1785. Many preparations exist, from the simple powdered leaves to very powerful extracts of special substances (glycosides) such as digitalin and digoxin.

The following are the most important:

Digitalis Tablets, B.P. (sometimes called *Digitalis folia*) 30-100 mg. ($\frac{1}{2}$ to $1\frac{1}{2}$ grains).

Digoxin tablets ('Lanoxin'), 0·25 to 1·0 milligram.

Digoxin injection, B.P., for intravenous use, 2 to 4 ml.

Digoxin for intramuscular injection, 1 ml.

Tincture of digitalis (*Tinctura digitalis*), 0·3-1 ml. (5 to 15 minims) repeated; 30 to 90 minims, single dose.

Nativelle's digitaline or digitoxin (granules), (0·1-1 mg.). $\frac{1}{600}$ to $\frac{1}{60}$ grain.

N.B.—1 grain of digitalis leaves and $\frac{1}{600}$ grain of Nativelle's digitalin are both approximately equivalent in effect to 10 minims of tincture of digitalis and digoxin, 0·25 mg.

D

## Methods of administration of digitalis

Treatment of atrial (auricular) fibrillation with digitalis may be divided into stages:

   (i) Initial doses or reduction of heart-rate to about 70.

  (ii) Maintenance doses.

 (iii) Urgent cases.

*Initial doses.* Provided no digitalis has been taken within two or three days, a full dose of digitalis tablets or digoxin is given.

*Maintenance doses.* These are adjusted to maintain the pulse and apex rate between 60 and 80 per minute. One rest day in seven during which the drug is omitted is often of value.

*Urgent cases.* In very urgent cases the most rapid results are obtained by giving digoxin; e.g. 1 milligram by mouth will slow the heart-rate in 6 to 8 hours. If necessary, 0·75 to 1·0 mg. may be given intravenously in 10 to 20 ml. of normal saline. The heart-rate begins to fall in 10 minutes and the maximum effect of the dose is apparent in less than 2 hours. Digoxin should not be given by subcutaneous injection.

## Notes on the administration of digitalis

1. It was formerly the practice to give digitalis in a mixture containing the tincture. This is most undesirable because unless the mixture is quite fresh, the potency of the tincture is partially destroyed by the water present and, if more than a few days old, it is unreliable in its results.

2. During the treatment of atrial fibrillation with digitalis both the apex-rate and the pulse-rate should be recorded.

3. The urinary output should be carefully measured.

4. Digitalis is not rapidly absorbed from the alimentary tract, the average dose requiring about 6 hours. There is, therefore, no advantage in giving the drug orally more often than six hourly.

5. The excretion of the drug is also slow and cumulative effects may be seen, hence the value of omitting the drug one day a week.

## Toxic symptoms

These may be due to over-dosage, cumulative effect or idiosyncrasy. They include:

(i) Undue slowness of the pulse, e.g. below 60.

(ii) Coupling of beats (*pulsus bigeminus*) and other cardiac irregularities.

(iii) Nausea and vomiting. Anorexia and diarrhœa may occur

(iv) Diminished urinary output.

(v) Alterations in the electrocardiogram.

### Other drugs of the digitalis group

These are very much less frequently employed than digitalis and are only useful when patients show intolerance to the latter drug. They include strophanthus, ouabain and lanatoside.

### Quinidine sulphate [(60-300 mg.) 1 to 5 grains]

This is a drug allied to quinine in composition. It acts directly on the heart-muscle and, in some cases, by reducing its conductive power is able to restore atrial fibrillation to normal rhythm, so that the impulse causing contraction of the heart again passes normally from the sino-atrial node over the atria to the atrio-ventricular node.

Quinidine is not suitable for use in all cases of atrial fibrillation and very careful selection is necessary. There are certain dangers in its use, including embolism and toxic symptoms such as diarrhœa, vomiting, skin rashes, convulsions and sudden death.

*Technique of administration.* A preliminary period of rest in bed with a course of digitalis therapy is generally advisable.

1st day: a test dose of 180 mg. (3 grains) is given.

2nd day (if no toxic symptoms are shown by the test dose): 360 mg. (6 grains) every 3 hours for 4 doses (total, 1·5 grams, 24 grains).

3rd day: 360 mg. (6 grains) every 3 hours for 5 doses (total, 2·0 grams, 30 grains).

4th to 7th days: This dosage is continued. If the drug is successful normal rhythm will be established within this period and may be maintained by a dose of 300 mg. (5 grains) once or twice a day.

It is also of value in the condition known as paroxysmal tachycardia, when small doses are given once or twice daily with a view to preventing the recurrence of the condition.

### Procainamide ('Pronestyl') (0·5 to 1 gram)

This is a synthetic substance having somewhat similar actions and uses to quinidine in paroxysmal tachycardia. It may be given orally or by very slow intravenous injection (up to 10 ml., and not exceeding 50 mg. per minute), during which a check on the blood pressure is maintained.

## CIRCULATORY STIMULANTS

Circulatory stimulants are drugs which are given to improve the circulation. They are generally employed in acute conditions such as shock, sudden heart failure in pneumonia, coronary thrombosis and allied conditions, asphyxia and collapse under anæsthesia, diabetic coma or coma due to poisoning with morphine, barbiturates and carbon monoxide.

They may be roughly classified into two main groups:

(i) Those which raise the blood-pressure by their action on the arteries (vaso-constrictors).

(ii) Those stimulating the heart indirectly via the nervous system.

(i) Injections of adrenaline and posterior pituitary extract (e.g. Pitressin) are examples of drugs which owe their value as circulatory stimulants to their effect on the arteries. Ephedrine by injection has a similar effect. They cause constriction of the arteries by stimulating the plain muscle in their walls to contract. The result of this general arterial constriction is a rise in blood-pressure.

**Noradrenaline** ('Levophed') is usually given in a slow intravenous drip, 4 ml. of a 1 in 1000 solution being added to 1 litre of saline (page 173). Its main use is when the blood pressure is low in surgical shock and after myocardial infraction.

(ii) **Mephentermine** ('Mephine') is used to raise blood pressure in cases of shock and severe collapse, not caused by hæmorrhage (e.g. coronary thrombosis). It may be given by intravenous or intramuscular injection in doses of up to

20 or 30 mg. at intervals until the systotic blood pressure is maintained at 100 mm. Hg.

(iii) The drugs of the second group cannot be regarded as pure cardiac stimulants because they act indirectly on the cardiac mechanism through the nervous system. The vaso-motor centre in the medulla is closely connected to the respiratory centre, which is also stimulated by these drugs. Further, a drug stimulating the respiratory centre, by in-creasing respiration, will increase the oxygen content of the blood and this will indirectly aid the circulation by improving the nutrition of the heart. They are, therefore, both cardiac and respiratory stimulants and are sometimes called *Analeptics*.

The drugs in this group include a large number of synthetic preparations, some of which are "official" and others of the proprietary type.

### Nikethamide ('Coramine', 'Anacardone')

This may be given by subcutaneous, intramuscular or intravenous injection. Oral administration is not effective. The usual dose is from 1 to 4 ml. of a 25% solution.

### Leptazol ('Cardiazol')

This has a similar action and may be administered in the same ways. Large doses are also given in order to produce convulsions in the treatment of certain types of mental disorder (schizophrenia).

**Methyl amphetamine** ('Methedrine') 10 to 30 mg. is given by intramuscular or intravenous injection as a circulatory stimulant for collapse and shock and to raise blood-pressure.

### Pholedrine Sulphate ('Veritol')

1 ml. of 2 per cent solution is given by intravenous or intramuscular injection.

## DRUGS ACTING ON THE ARTERIES

The drugs in this group, which lower blood-pressure by dilating the arteries, are called vasodilators. Advantage is taken of both these effects for different conditions, i.e. (i)

Drugs are sometimes used especially for their power of dilating the coronary arteries. (ii) They may be employed with the definite intention of lowering blood-pressure. (iii) They may be used for their action in dilating the peripheral arteries in the limbs.

Vaso-constrictors have already been mentioned, viz. adrenaline, ephedrine, posterior pituitary extract, etc.

## Drugs used to dilate the coronary arteries

### The nitrites and nitrates

These drugs are used especially in the treatment of angina pectoris, both in acute attacks and with a view to reducing their frequency. Their main action is to dilate the coronary arteries.

### Glyceryl trinitrate tablets [0·5 to 1 mg. ($\frac{1}{130}$-$\frac{1}{60}$ grain)]

This is the most important drug used in the treatment of angina pectoris, the pain of which is rapidly relieved. The tablets (*Tabellæ glycerylis trinitratis*) are placed under the tongue or chewed very slowly but not swallowed. The drug is absorbed by the mucous membrane of the mouth, but has little effect if it enters the stomach.

Its action is more prolonged than that of amyl nitrite (i.e. up to 15 minutes) and, in addition to its use during anginal attacks, it may be given in small doses at regular intervals in order to reduce their frequency. Tablets should not be kept for more than three months as they then lose their potency.

### Amyl nitrite capsules

This is a volatile liquid given by inhalation. It is supplied in glass capsules containing 0·18 ml. (3 minims), which are broken in a handkerchief and then inhaled. Its action in angina pectoris is rapid but brief. It also dilates the other arteries of the body, and this can be observed in the flushing of the face and felt in the throbbing of the head after inhalation. It is sometimes used to relieve biliary and renal colic and hiccough.

Octyl nitrite has a similar action.

**Erythrol tetranitrate,** 15 to 60 mg. ($\frac{1}{4}$ to 1 grain) and 'Mycardol' (pentaerythritol tetranitrate) are similar in use and action to glyceryl trinitrate.

**Khellin** is a vegetable drug which not only dilates the coronary arteries but also relaxes the spasm of the bronchi in asthma.

'Benecardin' is a preparation of Khellin.

## Drugs used to lower blood pressure (Hypotensive Drugs)

High blood pressure or hypertension is very common, especially with advancing years, but only in certain cases is it considered necessary to take steps to lower it.

At one time the operation of sympathectomy was carried out, more recently a number of drugs have been employed although none are always entirely satisfactory.

Some of these drugs act on the sympathetic and parasympathetic nerve ganglia and are referred to as *ganglion blocking agents*. The main effect of this action is to cause dilatation of the arterioles, thereby reducing peripheral resistance and, consequently, a lowering of the blood pressure.

Other nerve impulses transmitted through the ganglia may also be affected so that side-effects may occur. These include dry mouth, constipation and possibly paralytic ileus which is very dangerous. Impairment of visual accommodation, difficulty in micturition and even impotence may be noticed.

If the blood pressure is lowered too much, giddiness or faintness on assuming the erect posture may occur (postural hypotension). Others, such as Rauwolfia appear to act on higher centres of the central nervous system which control blood pressure.

**Hexamethonium:** dose 250-500 mg. by mouth.

25-50 mg. by subcutaneous or intramuscular injection.

This was one of the first of this type of drug to be used but has been replaced by more easily managed preparations.

Careful observation of the blood pressure both lying down and standing, before and after injection, is necessary until the appropriate maintenance dose has been ascertained.

Over-dosage may produce a severe fall in blood pressure which is treated with injections of methylamphetamine ('Methedrine') or adrenaline.

**Pentolinium tartrate** ('Ansolysen') is more potent than hexamethonium, is better absorbed from the gut, and has an action lasting up to twelve hours. Initial oral dose 20 mg. increased gradually up to 100 mg. if necessary. The sub-cutaneous dose is 3 mg.

**Mecamylamine** ('Inversine'), dose 5-25 mg., is a ganglion-blocking agent having powerful hypotensive properties. It is well absorbed by the alimentary tract and is given twice or three times daily in increasing doses until the desired effect is obtained.

*Guanethedine* ('Ismelin'), commencing with 10 mg. doses, appears to be one of the best hypotensive drugs.

**Reserpine** ('Serpasil'). This is an alkaloid obtained from the roots of an Indian plant, *Rauwolfia serpentina*. It is a less potent hypotensive drug than the ganglion-blocking agents and probably acts on the vaso-constrictor centre in the brain. Reserpine alone has little effect on the blood pressure but when combined with ganglion-blocking agents permits a smaller dose of these drugs to be given and, therefore, reduces side-effects. The average dose is 0·5 mg. daily.

It also has a general sedative action and may be used in larger doses in schizophrenia and other psychiatric conditions.

**Hydralazine** ('Apresoline') and 'Veriloid' are also used.

In the treatment of patients with hypertension any one of these drugs may be used alone or may be given in combination with one of the others, thereby reducing the necessary dose of each substance. In addition a sedative such as pheno-barbitone or sodium amytal may be used and in obese patients a reducing diet may be ordered.

It is important to remember that diuretics such as *chloro-thiazide* ('Saluric') and chlorthalidone ('Hygroton') increase considerably the effect of hypotensive drugs, the dose of which may have to be halved when they are given together.

## DRUGS USED FOR THEIR ACTION ON THE PERIPHERAL ARTERIES

There are a number of conditions similar to Raynaud's disease which are characterized by narrowing or spasm of the peripheral arteries followed by defective nutrition and, later, gangrene in the extremities. Pain in the muscles, especially on walking (intermittent claudication) is a common symptom.

**Tolazoline** ('Priscol'), is a substance which produces dilatation of the peripheral blood vessels and its effects resemble those of the operation of sympathectomy in conditions such as Raynaud's disease and peripheral arteriosclerosis. It is given by mouth in doses of 25 to 50 mg. (1 to 2 tablets) three times a day. Ampoules of the same strength are available for intramuscular or slow intravenous injection. It is usually avoided in patients who also suffer from peptic ulcer or coronary disease.

'Hexopal' is also an important vaso-dilator used in Raynaud's disease, threatened gangrene, chilblains and similar conditions.

Other drugs having a similar action include dibenyline, phentolamine ('Rogitine' and 'Ronicol').

### Anti-histamine drugs

Histamine is a substance which is liberated in the tissues especially in allergic conditions such as hay fever and urticaria and which has an action on the local circulation directly opposite to that of adrenaline. It has a powerful action in dilating capillaries, and may increase their permeability so that plasma escapes into the tissues producing local œdema such as is seen in urticaria.

There are a number of drugs which block the action of histamine known as the anti-histamines. They include:

| | | |
|---|---|---|
| 'Thephorin' | (Phenindamine) | 25 to 50 mg. |
| 'Phenergan' | (Promethazine) | 25 to 75 mg. |
| 'Benadryl' | (Diphenhydramine) | 50 mg. |
| 'Histantin' | (Chlorcyclazine) | 50 to 100 mg. |
| 'Antistin' | (Antazoline) | 100 mg. |
| 'Anthisan' | (Mepyramine) | 100 mg. |

They are given once, twice or three times a day according to their duration of action and should be taken after meals. They sometimes produce marked drowsiness and should not be taken before driving a car or undertaking work requiring special skill unless their precise effect on the individual is known.

In addition to their value in most allergic conditions, these drugs are also useful in paralysis agitans, travel sickness and for the itching of obstructive jaundice. They are also used in the form of ointments to relieve irritation in some skin conditions and insect bites but may themselves cause dermatitis in sensitive patients.

In severe anaphylactic shock an intravenous preparation may be used following a subcutaneous injection of adrenaline.

# CHAPTER 8

# DRUGS ACTING ON THE BLOOD

Blood consists of red corpuscles, white cells and blood platelets floating in plasma.

## THE RED CELLS

The *red corpuscles* or erythrocytes, which number 5,000,000 per cubic millimetre, are biconcave discs containing hæmoglobin. Hæmoglobin consists of a protein globin, combined with an iron-containing pigment called hæmatin. The red corpuscles are developed in the bone-marrow from large nucleated cells called megaloblasts, which as they mature become smaller in size and are called normoblasts. Normoblasts become filled with hæmoglobin, lose their nuclei and are then discharged as the fully developed erythrocytes into the general circulation.

In order that the megaloblast may develop into the normoblast, the special blood-forming or anti-anæmic factor is necessary. This is produced by the interaction of the intrinsic factor (of Castle) in the gastric juice with an extrinsic factor in the diet which is now known to be vitamin $B_{12}$ and which is stored in the liver. It is not certain whether the two factors actually combine, as originally suggested by Castle, or whether the intrinsic factor acts by aiding the absorption of the extrinsic factor (vitamin $B_{12}$) from the alimentary tract.

In order that sufficient hæmoglobin may be manufactured in the body to fill the normoblast and permit its development into the fully formed red corpuscle, there must be an adequate supply of iron. This is normally taken in the diet and absorbed from the alimentary tract.

In disease, the red corpuscles may either be defective (anæmia) or excessive in number (polycythæmia). Anæmia may be defined as a deficiency in the number of red corpuscles or in the amount of hæmoglobin, or both.

Anæmia may be due to:

Defective blood formation.
Excessive blood loss.
Excessive blood destruction.

## Drugs used for defective blood formation

### 1. Anæmia due to lack of anti-anæmic factor

Deficiency of anti-anæmic factor occurs in Addison's or pernicious anæmia, in the anæmia of sprue and similar rare types. It is due, in pernicious anæmia, to the absence of the intrinsic factor from the gastric juice, which means that anti-anæmic factor cannot be manufactured. The treatment therefore depends on supplying anti-anæmic factor, in the form of vitamin $B_{12}$, liver or stomach extracts.

### Vitamin $B_{12}$ and liver extracts

Fresh liver is now never used and vitamin $B_{12}$ has largely replaced liver extracts.

Both vitamin $B_{12}$ and liver extract may be given: (i) by intramuscular injection, which is the usual, more efficient and economical method (in very urgent cases intravenous injection is sometimes employed), or (ii) by mouth. Different preparations are available for each form of therapy. Treatment is divided into two stages:

1. The therapeutic stage, when large doses are employed until the blood-count has reached normal. Injections are given daily or two or three times a week.
2. The maintenance stage, which is continued indefinitely by injections every three or four weeks ("Depot dosage").

When the oral method is used vitamin $B_{12}$ or liver extract is given daily, the dosage being adapted to the stage of the treatment.

Vitamin $B_{12}$ (**Cyanocobalamin**). This is usually given by intramuscular injection in doses of 50 to 1000 micrograms. Preparations include 'Cytamen', 'Anacorbin', 'Distivit,' etc. For oral administration 'Biopar' tablets may be used. Liver extracts for **injection** having doses of 2 to 4 ml. include:

'Hepastab'. 'Anahæmin'. 'Pernæmon'.

With the "depot dosage system" employed in the maintenance stage, multiples of the above doses may be given.

### Stomach extracts

These, which are rarely used, are dry extracts of hog's stomach given by mouth and include the following proprietary preparations (dose 8 to 30 grams, ¼ to 1 ounce): 'Gastrexo', 'Pepsac', 'Ventriculin'.

**Folic Acid.** This is one of the factors in the vitamin B complex which, although it will restore the blood picture in pernicious anæmia to normal will not prevent the development of neurological complications. It should not, therefore be used in this condition.

It is, however, valuable in the treatment of anæmia in sprue, coeliac disease and the rare megalocytic anæmia of pregnancy. Dose: 5-20 mg. daily.

### 2. Defective hæmoglobin formation

Defective formation of hæmoglobin is due to lack of iron. This may result from a deficiency of iron in the diet or defective absorption of iron from the alimentary tract. It may also occur after loss of blood by hæmorrhage, when hæmoglobin is lost from the body in the red corpuscles and an additional quantity of iron is required for the manufacture of new supplies.

(1) **Iron is given by mouth, e.g.**

Ferrous sulphate (*Tab. ferri sulphatis co.*, N.F., 'Fersolate'), 200 mg. (3 grains).

Ferrous gluconate, 300 mg. (5 grains).

Ferric ammonium citrate (*Ferri et ammonii citras*), 2·4 grams (20 to 40 grains). This is given in mixture form but tends to blacken the teeth. It is less likely to produce gastric disturbances than some of the other preparations.

Ferrous carbonate or Blaud's pill or tablet (*Pilula ferri carbonatis*), 2 grams (5 to 30 grains).

(2) Various preparations of iron may be given by careful intravenous injections:

e.g. Saccharated iron oxide ('Ferrivenin').

These are specially prepared solutions which may cause soreness of the arm or phlebitis if they escape from the vein. Occasionally serious collapse may follow an injection. After an initial dose of 2·5 ml., 5 ml. (containing 100 mg.), or 10 ml. doses may be given daily or on alternate days until the required amount of iron has been administered, according to the formula

$$\frac{100 - \text{estimated hæmoglobin}}{100} \times 2500 \text{ mg.}$$

(3) 'Imferon' is an iron-dextran complex which may be given by intramuscular injection. The usual dose is 5 ml. When given by intramuscular injection, great care must be taken to see that none of the solution remains in the needle track. Otherwise some permanent staining of the skin may result. 'Jectofer' is another intramuscular iron preparation.

Other preparations containing iron, not used in the treatment of anæmia, but given as "tonics" (of doubtful value) are:

Parrish's Food (*Syrupus ferri phosphatis compositus*), 30-120 minims.

Easton's syrup (*Syrupus ferri phosphatis cum quinina et strychnina*) 30-60 minims.

## Excessive blood loss

In severe hæmorrhage there is loss of red corpuscles, hæmoglobin and fluid (plasma), and the ideal treatment is their replacement by blood transfusion. The loss of fluid, which is even more important than the loss of hæmoglobin, can also be made up by giving water by mouth, or saline by rectal, subcutaneous, intravenous and intraperitoneal infusions. Injections of Dextran and plasma transfusions are also of value.

Residual anæmia due to deficiency of hæmoglobin requires treatment with iron. Liver extract and vitamin $B_{12}$ are of no value in anæmia of this type because there is no deficiency of anti-anæmic factor.

## Excessive blood destruction

This is usually due to toxic processes and is treated by removing the cause, blood transfusion and iron administration.

## Excessive blood formation

In a disease known as polycythæmia (Osler's disease) in which the spleen is enlarged, and also in certain other circumstances, the number of red corpuscles may be considerably increased above the normal (up to 8 or 10 million per c.mm.). Symptoms are relieved by venesection, which is repeated as often as necessary. Radio-active Phosphorus ($P^{31}$) is the most effective treatment for this condition.

## THE WHITE CELLS

There are two important varieties of white cell, the leucocyte, having a granular protoplasm (granulocyte), and the lymphocyte. The former develop in the bone marrow, the latter in the lymphoid tissue (e.g. the lymph glands and spleen). The normal number of white cells in the blood is 6000 to 8000 per cubic millimetre, of which about 70 per cent are leucocytes and 30 per cent lymphocytes. If the total number of white cells is less than 5000 per c.mm. the condition is known as leucopœnia, if more than 10,000 per c.mm. it is called leucocytosis. Leukæmia is a disease in which very large numbers up to 100,000 or more are found. Mustine (Nitrogen mustard), Busulphan ('Myleran'), Chlorambucil ('Leukeran'), 'Colcemid', Aminopterin and Cortisone are drugs which may be used in the treatment of leukæmia. Their effect is uncertain and many cases are resistant. Side-effects may be unpleasant.

## Drugs producing leucopœnia

In addition to their reduction in diseases such as typhoid fever, the white cells, especially the polymorphonuclear leucocytes, may be seriously diminished (granulocytopœnia) or completely absent (agranulocytosis) as a result of the toxic action of certain drugs. These drugs are given for other purposes, but it is important to remember this dangerous effect in persons who show idiosyncrasy to them.

The most important drugs liable to produce severe leucopœnia (granulocytopœnia or agranulocytosis) are:

| Thiouracil and its | Chloramphenicol. |
| derivatives. | Tridione. |
| The sulphonamides. | Mesontoin. |
| Amidopyrine. | Phenylbutazone ('Butazolidine'). |
| Gold salts. | Radio-active substances. |

## Drugs producing leucocytosis

The only condition in which an attempt has been made to increase the number of leucocytes by giving drugs is the one just mentioned, viz. granulocytopœnia. The substance employed is pentose nucleotide. The average dose is 15 ml. twice daily for several days by intra-muscular injection but its effect is doubtful. Antibiotics are given to prevent infection.

## THE VOLUME OF THE BLOOD

The total volume of the blood is made up by the plasma and the blood-cells. It may be decreased by loss of both in severe hæmorrhage. The fluid portion alone may be diminished in states of dehydration due to excessive fluid loss from the tissues in severe vomiting, diarrhœa, diabetic coma, severe burns and insufficient fluid intake, i.e. the plasma becomes more concentrated.

The treatment of these conditions necessitates the replacement of fluid by one of the following means:

(i) Blood transfusion, indicated when both plasma and red corpuscles have been lost by hæmorrhage.

(ii) Plasma transfusion, especially in cases of shock but also of value after hæmorrhage.

(iii) Dextran by intravenous injection.

(iv) Normal saline by rectal, subcutaneous, intravenous or intraperitoneal injection in any case of fluid loss.

(v) Normal saline with glucose by rectal or intravenous injection.

(vi) Water or half-strength normal saline by mouth.

### Blood transfusion

The main indications are:

I. Severe hæmorrhage—

(a) Accidents.        (b) Before and after operation.

(c) Conditions such as hæmatemesis, abortion, and post-partum hæmorrhage.

II. Medical conditions—

    (*a*) Severe hypochromic anæmia.
    (*b*) Some cases of septicæmia.
    (*c*) Hæmophilia.
    (*d*) Occasionally in pernicious anæmia.

It has been found that, for purposes of blood transfusion, individuals may be divided into four groups, and it is only when they belong to the same group that their bloods will mix properly. If blood from the wrong group is transfused the red cells in it are destroyed with very serious and often fatal results to the recipient. It is, therefore, most important to discover the group to which the patient belongs and to select a suitable donor. It is also necessary to test the blood for Rhesus factor (Rh.)

In view of the danger to life if blood of the wrong group is given, any nurse handling bottles of blood for transfusion must be particularly careful to see that they reach the right patient, as confusion can occur, especially if more than one transfusion is going on at the same time. Before each bottle is given its label and group should be checked by two persons and compared with the known group of the patient.

BLOOD GROUPS

| Moss | International | Percentage of Persons |
|:----:|:------------:|:---------------------:|
| I | AB | 5 |
| II | A | 40 |
| III | B | 10 |
| IV | O | 45 |

There is an exception to this rule concerning what are called group O or IV donors. In most instances their blood may be given to any patient without causing ill effects, and they are, therefore, referred to as universal donors, but even with these donors a preliminary test must be made to ensure compatibility.

As a rule, 500 to 1000 ml. (about 1 to 2 pints) of blood are given as a single transfusion.

The continuous drip method is generally used, and by this means as much as 4 to 5 pints may be given over a period of 24 hours at the rate of about 40 drops a minute.

The basis of modern blood-transfusion technique is to collect blood from a donor into a vacuum bottle containing a special solution of sodium citrate to prevent clotting. Blood thus obtained can be stored in a cold place for about two weeks.

### Packed cell transfusion

"Concentrated human red blood corpuscles" is whole human blood from which 40 per cent of the plasma has been removed. This form of transfusion may be used in certain cases of anæmia when it is especially desirable to raise the hæmoglobin rapidly without introducing a large amount of fluid into the circulation.

### Plasma transfusion

Plasma will keep longer than citrated blood containing red cells and therefore plasma may be withdrawn from citrated blood after the red corpuscles have fallen by sedimentation to the bottom of the collecting bottle, and stored for a long period.

Plasma is of great value in restoring the blood volume in cases of shock. It may also be stored in dry form. Dry plasma is rendered suitable for intravenous injection by dissolving 20 grams in 500 ml. of sterile 5 per cent dextrose in distilled water and using it at once.

Human blood serum may also be used in the same way and can be stored in dry form.

### SALINE SOLUTIONS

The blood and tissue fluids normally contain a more or less constant concentration of various salts, and one of the functions of the kidneys is to keep this at a steady level. If the concentration of salts in the blood is increased there will be a passage of fluid from the tissues to the blood until the salt concentration of both is again equal (i.e. a passage from the weaker to the stronger to produce equality).

The effect produced by this concentration of salts (and other substances) is called osmotic pressure, and, in the example just given, the osmotic pressure in the blood would be greater than that in the tissues and, as a result, water would be withdrawn from the latter until the osmotic pressures of the blood and tissue fluids were equal.

Solutions of salts and other substances are frequently injected into the blood-stream for various therapeutic purposes, or they may be applied externally to wounds, etc. Depending on their strength (concentration) such solutions may have the same osmotic pressure as the blood, when they are said to be isotonic (iso = equal). Their strength may be less than that of the blood and, if injected, would have a weakening or diluting effect (hypotonic), or they may be stronger solutions (hypertonic). Hypotonic solutions are not often used in therapeutics.

### Normal or isotonic saline

The term saline used in this connection refers to a solution of sodium chloride or common salt, and normal saline is a sterile solution of sodium chloride in water having a strength of 0·9 per cent.

The concentration of sodium chloride being the same as that of the various salts in the blood, when normal saline is injected intravenously it does not affect the balance which exists between the blood and tissue fluids—unless this is already abnormal and the saline is given to restore the balance to normal.

### Hypertonic saline

This is a solution of sodium chloride in water exceeding the strength of normal saline (0·9 per cent). Various concentrations are employed according to the purposes for which they are needed.

When given by intravenous injection, the effect will be to raise the salt concentration in the blood so that it is higher than that in the tissues. The result of this is the withdrawal of fluid from the tissues.

For example, 30 ml. of 30 per cent saline (or 50 ml. of 15 per cent) may be injected intravenously in cases of raised intracranial pressure. The effect is withdrawal of fluid from the brain into the blood. In consequence the brain shrinks in size, thus lowering the tension within the cranium. The more usual practice, however, is to inject 500 ml. of 50 per cent sucrose. A similar effect is produced more slowly by the rectal injection of hypertonic magnesium sulphate solution (6 ounces of 25 per cent).

Hypertonic saline is also applied as a wound dressing and by its hypertonic action promotes the flow of tissue fluids into the wound.

### Glucose-saline solution (*Liquor dextrosi et sodii chloridi,* B.P.C.)

This consists of 5 per cent glucose and 0·9 per cent sodium chloride. It is therefore slightly hypertonic, but the glucose is rapidly absorbed after injection and from a practical point of view the solution may be regarded as having an isotonic effect.

Hypertonic glucose solutions up to 25 per cent are sometimes used for special purposes.

One to two litres of a sterile solution of **Dextran** (6 per cent) in normal saline is sometimes given intravenously in cases of severe hæmorrhage when blood is not available for transfusion and also in cases of shock. It is made up to have the same osmotic pressure as blood. Its main effect is to increase the blood volume and has the advantage over normal saline that it is not so rapidly excreted and, therefore, exercises its action for a longer period after injection.

Gum acacia (6 per cent) has been similarly employed.

**Hartmann's solution** (*Injectio sodii lactatis composita,* B.P.) may be given orally, subcutaneously or intravenously in the treatment of gastro-enteritis in children and other conditions when acidosis is present. It contains lactic acid and the chlorides of sodium, potassium and calcium.

**Hyaluronidase ('Hyalase').** This is an enzyme found in various animal tissues which may be described as a "spreading factor". That is to say, it increases the permeability of the capillaries and tissues so that substances injected into the latter can be more easily dispersed and more rapidly absorbed into the blood-stream.

This is of particular value when intravenous therapy is impossible or undesirable. 'Hyaluronidase' has many uses, in particular the administration of subcutaneous saline (e.g. in infants) and for pyelograms when a vein cannot be used. 1 ml., containing 1000 units in distilled water, is injected into the site of the proposed infusion. The solution must be freshly prepared.

## The Anti-coagulant Drugs

Substances such as potassium citrate which can prevent clotting when added to blood after it has been withdrawn from the body have already been mentioned (page 59).

The ability of blood to clot is one of Nature's processes which protects the individual against excessive bleeding as a result of injury.

The actual mechanism is a complicated one and involves the interaction of a number of substances present in the blood, the liver and the tissues. It may be briefly simplified in the following way:

1. Blood = $\begin{cases} \text{Corpuscles} \\ + \\ \text{Plasma} = \end{cases}$ $\begin{cases} \text{Fibrin} \\ + \\ \text{Serum} \end{cases}$ = Clot.

2. (*a*) Prothrombin + thrombokinase (thromboplastin) + Calcium→thrombin.

   (*b*) Thrombin + fibinogen→Clot.

Clotting of blood within the blood vessels, or thrombosis, is not an uncommon pathological condition. There are drugs which can be given internally which prevent or diminish the risk of clotting within the body. These are referred to as anti-coagulants and are of two main types:

    1. Heparin.
    2. The Coumarin group ('Dindevan', 'Sinthrome').

The two groups of drugs act at different stages of the clotting process.

(1) **Heparin** is an anti-coagulant substance prepared from liver. It acts rapidly and is soon eliminated from the system. It is usually given by intravenous injection in doses of 5,000 to 10,000 units every six hours. In order to facilitate this a special needle with a non-leaking diaphragm may be left in the vein if desired, or 1,000 units per hour may be given in a saline drip.

Heparin may be given by intramuscular injection, using a very fine needle, but there is risk of local hæmatoma formation. It is absorbed slowly and its action is less reliable when given by this route. If the administration of Heparin is prolonged, the dosage is controlled by estimating the clotting time of the blood.

*Overdosage.* The antidote to over dosage is the intravenous injection of protamine sulphate, 50 mg. of which will neutralize the effect of 5,000 units of Heparin. A blood transfusion may also be given.

(2) **'Dindevan', 'Sinthrome'.** These substances which belong to the coumarin group of drugs, differ from each other somewhat in chemical composition but all act by preventing the formation of prothrombin in the liver. Thus they take some time to act since all the prothrombin present in the blood must first be used up, which takes about twenty-four hours. They are given by mouth.

'Dicoumarol' and 'Tromexan' are no longer used.

**Phenindione.** ('Dindevan') is given in doses of 100 mg. followed by 50 mg. once or twice daily.

**Nicoumalone.** ('Sinthrome') is supplied in 4 mg. tablets. The average dose is: 1st day 20-28 mg., 2nd day 16-24 mg., 3rd and subsequent days 4-12 mg.

Since these drugs take about a day before they act, it is a common practice to commence anti-coagulant therapy with Heparin for twenty-four hours, during which the first tablets of 'Dindevan' or 'Sinthrome' are also given. Their dosage is controlled by estimations of the blood prothrombin level which is usually reduced to about 40 per cent.

*Overdosage* will result in a prothrombin level of below 30 per cent and may be followed by bleeding into the skin and mucous membranes (purpura), the presence of red cells in the urine (hæmaturia), vaginal hæmorrhage or excessive hæmorrhage from recent wounds or operation sites. The treatment is to stop the drug at once and to give blood transfusions and intravenous vitamin $K_1$. (Ordinary water-soluble vitamin K is ineffective.)

Anti-coagulants are used in the treatment of coronary artery thrombosis, pulmonary embolism and thrombosis of veins in the limbs, etc. They do not dissolve clot once it has formed, but prevent either the development of, or extension of, thrombosis.

# CHAPTER 9

# DRUGS ACTING ON THE RESPIRATORY SYSTEM

For purposes of therapeutics it is convenient to consider separately the lower respiratory tract, consisting of the trachea, bronchi and alveoli of the lungs; and the upper respiratory tract which includes the nose, pharynx and larynx.

The object of respiration is the interchange of gases between the blood and the atmosphere, oxygen being absorbed and carbon dioxide (and water) being excreted by the lungs.

The rate and depth of respiration is controlled by the respiratory centre in the medulla oblongata in such a way that the concentration of oxygen and carbon dioxide in the blood is normally kept constant. This is done in the following way: The respiratory centre is especially sensitive to the amount of carbon dioxide in the blood. If this rises above the normal (e.g. as a result of exercise) the respiratory centre is stimulated so that the rate and depth of respiration are increased. The increase in the respiratory movements results in a greater intake of oxygen and an increased excretion of carbon dioxide, so that the concentration of the latter in the blood tends to fall to normal once more.

Other substances may also influence the respiratory centre. They may produce similar stimulation, with increased movements, or alternatively they may depress the centre so that breathing becomes slower and shallower.

The respiratory tract is lined with ciliated epithelium, the cells of which also secrete mucus. The bronchioles have plain muscle-fibres in their walls.

There are two troublesome symptoms which occur in a number of disorders affecting the respiratory system viz.:

1. Cough.

2. Bronchospasm.

A cough is a reflex act having a cough centre in the medulla. The stimulus provoking a cough may arise from irritation or inflammation in the pharynx, larynx, trachea, bronchi, lungs or pleura. It may be:

(a) dry and unproductive.

(b) loose and with sputum.

(a) Sometimes it is desirable to suppress a distressing dry cough by means of a sedative linctus containing drugs which depress the cough reflex by acting on the centre.

(b) Expectorant drugs may be needed to loosen sticky sputum.

## DRUGS STIMULATING THE RESPIRATORY CENTRE

It has already been seen that cardiac and respiratory stimulants (analeptics) are closely allied and that an increase in respiration has a beneficial effect on the heart by increasing its oxygen supply (page 93). The stimulants of the respiratory centre are, therefore, used to counteract its depression in cases of heart failure, also in various types of poisoning, during anæsthesia and other conditions in which respiratory failure may be evident. They include:

| | |
|---|---|
| Nikethamide ('Coramine') | Nalorphine ('Lethidrone') |
| Leptazol ('Cardiazol') | Strychnine |
| Aminophylline (page 120) | Caffeine |
| Bemegride ('Megimide') | Lobeline |
| Picrotoxin (page 149) | Carbon dioxide |

### Lobeline

This is the alkaloid obtained from lobelia. It is a powerful respiratory stimulant and is used in various emergencies, including coal gas and morphine poisoning. Adult dose, up to 20 mg. ($\frac{1}{3}$ grain).

It is also used for infants with asphyxia neonatorum, injections of 3 mg. ($\frac{1}{20}$ grain) being given into the umbilical vein.

### Carbon dioxide

Carbon dioxide ($CO_2$) is a colourless gas which plays a number of important parts in the economy of Nature. It is an oxide of the element carbon and is produced when carbon is burnt in the presence of sufficient oxygen. It must not be confused with carbon monoxide (CO), a very poisonous oxide of carbon, which is present in large amount in domestic coal gas.

Carbon dioxide is present in the atmospheric air, i.e. inspired air (0·04 per cent), and in expired air (4 per cent). It is soluble in water. In the manufacture of "soda water", the gas is dissolved in water under pressure. Owing to the escape of carbon dioxide the solution effervesces when the pressure is withdrawn. Beer, champagne and effervescing mineral waters ("aerated waters") also give off carbon dioxide.

It can be compressed by pumping it into steel cylinders and, by special methods, can be converted into a solid, soft, snow-like substance, "carbon dioxide snow", which only remains solid at a very low temperature.

The main use of carbon dioxide is as a respiratory stimulant. Mixtures containing 5 to 10 per cent of carbon dioxide with oxygen are administered by inhalation. The additional concentration of carbon dioxide thus produced in the lungs leads to an increase in the amount in the blood. The respiratory centre is, therefore, stimulated so that respiration is increased in frequency and depth.

It is employed particularly during general anæsthesia, when respiration is shallow in order to increase its depth; and also when the administration has ceased, with a view to increasing the amount of anæsthetic excreted by the lungs and so hastening the recovery of consciousness.

It is also of value in poisoning by substances which depress the respiratory centre such as morphine, opium and barbiturates.

It is useful in helping the expansion of the lungs after any portion has been collapsed, e.g. by the pressure of a pleural effusion, and after abdominal operations when the action of the diaphragm may have been impaired.

A solution of carbon dioxide in water, e.g. "soda water", has a mildly stimulating effect on the mucous membrane of the stomach, improving the appetite and causing a feeling of well-being. Effervescing waters are therefore of value in cases of gastric catarrh. The increased blood-supply to the mucous membrane caused by this stimulating effect hastens the absorption of water and other substances which accounts for the rapid absorption of alcohol from sparkling wines such as champagne and may explain their exceptionally exhilarating effect.

In solid form, *"carbon dioxide snow"*, which can be produced in the shape of a cone or pencil, is applied to the skin in the treatment of nævi, moles, warts, etc., on which it has a freezing action. If contact is too prolonged blister formation may ensue.

## Oxygen

Although not a respiratory stimulant, oxygen may be conveniently considered here on account of its use in cases of respiratory failure.

The atmosphere (inspired air) contains 20 per cent oxygen and the expired air 16 per cent. The 4 per cent oxygen absorbed via the alveoli of the lungs into the blood is conveyed in the red corpuscles to the tissues as oxyhæmoglobin.

The amount of oxygen carried to the tissues may be **decreased** by (*a*) diseases of the lungs and disorders of the pulmonary circulation, whereby the blood fails to acquire sufficient oxygen during its passage through the lungs.

(*b*) General circulatory failure with stagnation of venous blood in the peripheral parts.

(*c*) Deficiency in the oxygen-carrying power of the blood due to decrease in the amount of hæmoglobin or red corpuscles, i.e. anæmia.

(*d*) Defective oxygen-carrying power of hæmoglobin by its conversion into carboxyhæmoglobin in coal gas (carbon monoxide) poisoning.

The amount of oxygen in the blood can only be *increased* by increasing the amount of oxygen in the alveolar air. This may be done by the administration of oxygen by inhalation.

Oxygen may be given in the following ways:

1. The oxygen tent, the ideal method especially for children.

2. The B.L.B. mask.

3. A light-weight polythene bag or nasal catheter.

The ideal administration of oxygen by any method requires some sort of flow meter with a fine adjustment valve in order that economical and efficient use may be obtained. The amount of oxygen usually required is 4 to 6 litres per minute.

In many hospitals oxygen is piped to each bedside from a central supply.

(a) A 100 cubic foot oxygen cylinder with a rate of flow of 4 litres per minute will last about 12 hours.

(b) No oil or lubricant must be put on the high-pressure valves as this may cause fire.

(c) Under no circumstances should matches or cigarettes be brought near to a patient having oxygen.

Oxygen given by the tube and funnel method does not raise the oxygen content of the alveolar air sufficiently to have any effect. It therefore has no other use than impressing anxious relatives that something is being done, and is a waste of oxygen.

Passing oxygen through water in a Woulf's bottle at a rate at which bubbles can just be counted supplies less than 0·5 litre per minute. This is insufficient to produce any really beneficial effect.

The greatest care must be taken to discriminate between (a) pure oxygen and (b) oxygen and carbon dioxide mixtures. The latter should only be used when specially ordered.

Particular care is also necessary not to administer oxygen for too long or in too great a concentration to premature and new-born infants. Blindness due to a condition known as retrolental fibroplasia may be caused by excess.

## DRUGS WHICH DEPRESS THE RESPIRATORY CENTRE

There are a number of drugs which slow the rate and diminish the depth of respiration. They are not, however, employed therapeutically to produce this result and this action must be regarded as a side effect of their uses for other purposes for example:

All general anæsthetics.

Alcohol.

Barbiturates.

Chloral and other hypnotics in toxic doses.

## Cough-suppressants

Drugs which reduce the excitability of the respiratory centre and are thereby effective in diminishing a dry and unproductive cough include:

| | |
|---|---|
| Morphine and opium | Methadone ('Physeptone') |
| Diamorphine (Heroin) | Pholcodine ('Ethnine' etc.) |
| Codeine | |

These drugs are often employed in various linctuses which are made up with syrup. The dose is usually 2 to 4 ml. (60 to 120 minims).

| | |
|---|---|
| *Linctus scillæ opiatus* | *Linctus methadoni* |
| *Linctus codeinæ* | *Linctus pholcodine* |

Other preparations include, Narcotine linctus, 'Toclase', 'Taoryl', 'Sedulon', and 'Tusana'. There are in fact an enormous number of proprietary cough medicines the respective merits of which are difficult to compare.

Sucking a sweet or medicated lozenge (e.g. liquorice) will often help a troublesome cough.

# DRUGS AFFECTING BRONCHIAL SECRETION
## Expectorants

An expectorant may be defined as a drug which aids the expulsion of mucus from the respiratory tract either by increasing its secretion or by "loosening" it so that it becomes less tenacious and sticky.

Recent research indicates that many of the drugs which were formerly regarded as increasing the amount of mucus secreted, probably do not act in this way and that they owe their usefulness to their "loosening" effect, which makes expectoration of sputum easier. There is little doubt, however, that in practice the so-called cough mixture is appreciated by the patient and that it relieves his symptoms.

In smaller doses, a number of emetic drugs (see page 64), such as ipecacuanha act as expectorants. Potassium iodide in addition to other effects, also appears to increase and loosen secretion from the respiratory mucous membrane. It will be remembered that one of the symptoms of "iodism" is that of a common cold in which the flow of mucus from the nose and bronchi is increased (page 29).

The following are among the important expectorants and one or more are often combined in cough mixtures:

Ammonium bicarbonate       Senega
Ipecacuanha                Squill
Potassium iodide

e.g. *Mituræ ammoniæs et ipecacuanhæ*, known also as Mistura Expectorans.

### Squill (*Scilla*)

In addition to its effect on the heart which, in appropriate doses, is similar to that of digitalis, squill also acts as an expectorant by reason of its irritating effect on the bronchial mucous membrane. It is, therefore, more suited to cases of chronic than of acute bronchitis. It is an irritating drug and in large doses acts as a gastro-intestinal irritant and irritant to the kidneys.

### Senega

This is usually prescribed in the form of mixtures containing:
Infusion of senega (*Infusum senegæ*), 30 ml. ($\frac{1}{2}$ to 1 ounce).

Bronchial secretion may be loosened and expectoration helped by the following:

(*a*) Sodium chloride mixture (*Mist. sodii. chlor. co.*) taken in hot water.

(*b*) Steam inhalations to which may be added Benzoin (Friar's balsam) inhalation.

(*c*) Aerosols containing detergents, e.g. 'Alevair', and similar preparations which are sometimes called "mucolytics".

## Anti-expectorants

By this term is meant drugs which reduce bronchial secretion; the most important being belladonna and its alkaloid, atropine. Stramonium has a similar effect. Atropine is used before general anæsthetics, especially ether, in order to prevent excessive bronchial secretion. It is also given in cases of pulmonary œdema (see also page 177).

## Antispasmodics

Severe spasm of the bronchioles occurs in asthma and is due to contraction of the plain muscle fibres in their walls. Some bronchial spasm may also occur in bronchitis. The following drugs by their action on the bronchial muscle-fibres relax the spasm:

Adrenaline: Subcutaneous injection of 1 in 1000 solution (page 173) in doses up to 1 ml. (3 to 15 minims), depending on the severity and duration of the spasm.

Isoprenaline: is a substance having a similar action to adrenaline. It may be used as a 20 mg. tablet which is allowed to dissolve under the tongue and also in nasal sprays. Proprietary preparations include 'Aleudrin', 'Neo-drenal' and 'Neo-Epinine'.

Ephedrine (*Ephedrinæ hydrochloridum*): 100 mg. ($\frac{1}{4}$ to $1\frac{1}{2}$ grains) may be given by mouth or by injection.

Ammophylline ⎫ These drugs are all antispasmodics and are
Atropine ⎬ sometimes used for the relief of asthma
Stramonium ⎬ and bronchitis associated with bronchial
Lobelia ⎭ spasm.

Steroid preparations may be required in status asthmaticus which fails to respond to other remedies.

### Stramonium

In large doses, stramonium has an effect on the nervous system which makes it of value in reducing the muscular rigidity present in Parkinsonism (paralysis agitans). When very large doses are given they have a similar effect to atropine and diminish bronchial secretion and make the mouth dry. To counteract this, pilocarpine, 6 mg. ($\frac{1}{10}$ grain), is administered at the same time. Preparation:

Tincture of stramonium (*Tinctura stramonii*), 2 ml. (5 to 30 minims).

In Parkinsonism the dose may be gradually increased to 4 ml. (60 minims) or more.

### Lobelia

This may be combined with stramonium in cough mixtures. The important alkaloid lobeline (page 113), which stimulates the respiratory centre, is obtained from lobelia.

**Aminophylline** ('Cardophyllin' or Theophylline with Ethy-
lenediamine).

This drug has a number of actions. It acts on the heart
and reduces venous pressure in congestive heart failure. It is
also helpful in angina pectoris. Bronchospasm is relieved,
hence it is often employed in the treatment of bronchial
asthma, especially if there has been no relief from adrenaline
or isoprenaline. It is also of value in nocturnal dyspnœa in
heart disease ("cardiac asthma") when one or two suppositories
may be given at night. Intravenous aminophylline will often
abolish Cheyne-Stokes breathing. It also has a mild diuretic
action. It may be given by mouth (up to 500 mg.), suppository,
or slow intravenous injection (250 mg. in 10 ml.). Intramuscular injection is often painful.

'Choledyl' (oxytriphylline). This drug has an action
similar to aminophylline but is less irritating to the stomach.
Dose: 100-400 mg.

**Theophylline Sodium Glycinate** ('Englate') available in
tablets and as a linctus is useful for mild bronchospasm.

Both 'Choledyl' and 'Englate' are very useful drugs in
acute or chronic bronchitis when the chest is wheezy.

### Pulmonary antiseptics

Drugs such as cresote and guaiacol which were formerly
used as pulmonary antiseptics have now been replaced by
sulphonamides, penicillin and other antibiotics such as tetracycline which are selected according to the sensitivity of the
organisms found in the sputum in bronchitis, pneumonia,
lung abscess and bronchiectasis.

### Drugs used in radiography of the chest

Iodized oil, i.e. 'Lipiodol' and similar preparations (page
45) are introduced into the trachea from which, by adjusting
the position of the patient, they run into the bronchi of either
lung. The following methods may be employed: (i) A nasal
catheter is passed so that its end over-hangs the larynx and the
oil drops down. (ii) The oil is dropped from a special syringe
over the back of the tongue. (iii) It is injected into the trachea

through the crico-thyroid membrane after local anæsthesia. General anæsthesia may be needed for children.

Iodized oil is opaque to X-rays and is of value in the diagnosis of bronchiectasis, lung abscess and new growth of the lung.

'Dionosil' (propyliodone) is a watery solution which can be used to obtain bronchograms either by the cricothyroid route or by direct injection through an endotracheal tube. About 16 ml. are required for each lung in an adult. It has the advantage of not remaining for long periods in the bronchi and alveoli.

## DRUGS ACTING ON THE NOSE AND NASAL SINUSES

While it is not possible to give in detail all the drugs which are employed in affections of the nose, the following are the most important methods of application.

### Nasal Drops (naristillæ)

The most useful are Ephedrine nasal drops which have a vaso-constricting action and thereby help to shrink swollen and congested mucous membrane. They are of value in hay fever, sinusitis and also in acute otitis media where they decongest the mucous membrane around the opening of the Eustachian tube and allow drainage from the middle ear.

Oily solutions should not be instilled into the nose as they interfere with the action of cilia.

Drops should be instilled with the patient lying down with the head extended and breathing through the mouth.

Many proprietary nasal decongestants are available, e.g. 'Endrine', 'Neophryn', 'Privine'.

### Nasal douches (Collunaria)

Various solutions including saline, boric acid and alkaline lotions are employed for cleansing the nose of copious discharge and crusts.

They are best given with a douche can or funnel attached to an appropriate length of rubber tubing. The height of the can should not be more than 12 inches above the patient's

E

head. During the procedure the patient should be instructed to breathe heavily through the mouth.

The use of the Higginson syringe is most undesirable on account of the dangerously high pressure which can be obtained. Fluid may thus be forced into the middle ear via the Eustachian tube, causing a spread of infection.

Sniffing solutions into the nasal cavity is also inadvisable and may be followed by headache.

### Nasal sprays (*Nebulæ*)

Watery solutions are employed and sprayed into the nasal cavities by an appropriate atomizer or used as nasal drops.

Ephedrine, adrenaline, and menthol are the drugs most frequently used for catarrhal affections of the nose and for nasal sinusitis.

### Inhalations

Inhalations of menthol, 120 mg., 2 grains (4 or 5 small crystals), or compound tincture of benzoin (*Tinctura benzoini composita*—Friar's balsam), 4 ml. (60 minims) to 1 pint of boiling water, are commonly employed. They are of value in sinusitis, acute nasal catarrh, laryngitis, tracheitis and bronchitis.

### Insufflations and snuffs

These are occasionally employed, a special powder insufflator being used in some cases.

e.g. Orthocaine ('Orthoform') or benzocaine ('Anæsthesin') for pain.

Menthol snuff for nasal catarrh.

Posterior pituitary snuff ('Disipidin') for diabetes insipidus.

### Local anæsthetics

Injections of Procaine ('Novocain'), $\frac{1}{2}$ per cent, with a few drops of adrenaline, 1 in 1000, may be used.

Cocaine (5 to 10 per cent), which is never injected, may be used to produce local anæsthesia by plugging the nasal cavity with strips of $\frac{1}{2}$-inch gauze soaked in the solution.

Cocaine ointment may also be applied on a wool-coated probe.

'Decicain' (amethocaine), 2 per cent, is sometimes used instead of cocaine. Amethocaine has even been made into "Lollipops" for use before bronchoscopy!

### Caustics

Chromic acid, trichloracetic acid, silver nitrate or the electric cautery may be applied to ulcers in the nasal mucous membrane; or to a bleeding-point to stop epistaxis.

## DRUGS APPLIED TO THE LARYNX

Various drugs are applied to the larynx by inhalations, insufflations and sprays.

### Inhalations

Menthol and Friar's balsam are used as in the treatment of nasal conditions.

### Insufflations

Insufflations of anæsthetic powders are employed for the relief of pain, especially in tuberculous laryngitis, using Leduc's tube. About 250 mg. (4 grains) of orthocaine ('Orthoform') or benzocaine ('Anæsthesin') are insufflated 10 minutes before meals. Leduc's auto-insufflator consists of a glass tube bent at right angles at one end. This end is introduced well into the mouth to reach the pharynx. The other end rests on a saucer or suitable receptacle containing the powder. The patient closes the lips round the tube and takes several sharp inspirations which draw the powder into the larynx.

### Sprays

Sprays containing menthol, camphor and 'Chloretone' may be used for laryngitis. Lignocaine, 2 ml. of a 4 per cent solution, may be sprayed onto the larynx after the pharynx has been rendered insensitive by sucking a lignocaine lozenge containing 150 mg. in order to produce anæsthesia.

# CHAPTER 10

# DRUGS ACTING ON THE URINARY SYSTEM

The urinary system is formed by the kidneys, ureters, bladder and urethra. The kidneys are excretory glands and consist of cortex and medulla which are made up of Malpighian bodies and tubules. The ureter, its upper expanded part of the pelvis, the bladder and urethra form the ducts and reservoir via which the urine reaches the exterior.

The processes employed by the kidneys in the formation of urine are: 1. Filtration of water and salts through the Malpighian bodies. 2. Secretion of various substances by the tubules. 3. Absorption of water and substances excreted by the first two processes but required by the body to maintain the composition of the blood at a constant level.

The primary function of the kidneys is to keep the composition of the blood constant by:

(i) The excretion of water.

(ii) The excretion of the end products of protein metabolism.

(iii) The excretion of salts.

(iv) The excretion of drugs, toxins and chemical substances which may be harmful.

The kidneys are therefore of great importance in dealing with the subject of drugs. Many drugs given internally by mouth or injection, are excreted by the kidneys either in their original form or else changed by chemical action in the body (e.g. by the liver).

Some of these drugs have no effect on the urinary tract; others have a beneficial action in certain conditions and are given for this action. Finally, some have a harmful effect, especially when used in toxic doses, and may produce serious urinary symptoms such as hæmaturia.

## Diseases of the urinary tract

These include congenital abnormalities, traumatic and mechanical conditions, acute or chronic inflammation of the kidneys (nephritis), of the pelvis (pyelitis), of the bladder (cystitis), and of the urethra (urethritis), tuberculosis and new growths. Abnormal products of metabolism may also be excreted in the urine. Medical treatment may be required for many of these conditions. Further, it may be necessary to modify the excretory functions of the kidneys in order to relieve symptoms caused by disease of other organs, e.g. the removal of fluid in cases of œdema.

# DRUGS INCREASING THE OUTPUT OF URINE (DIURETICS)

A diuretic is a substance which increases the output of urine.

The amount of urine normally excreted depends on three factors:

(i) The fluid intake.

(ii) The fluid lost by the evaporation of sweat.

(iii) The amount lost via the bowel.

The most obvious physiological diuretic is water. In many cases, when the kidneys are normal this is the most suitable method of producing an increased urinary flow. On the other hand, diuretics are given in order to get rid of surplus fluid already present in the body, i.e. œdema. This occurs when water and salt are retained in the body particularly in the following conditions:

(a) congestive heart failure, (b) pulmonary œdema and congestion, (c) ascites in cirrhosis of the liver, (d) certain types of chronic nephritis.

The processes employed by the kidneys in the formation of urine have already been mentioned. A diuretic may act in one of the following ways:

(i) Increasing the filtration of water and salts through the Malpighian bodies by generally improving the blood supply to the kidneys. Blood transfusion and saline infusions will do this in cases of surgical shock and dehydration. Digitalis will improve the renal circulation in cardiac failure, especially when due to atrial fibrillation.

(ii) By preventing the reabsorption of water in the renal tubules, e.g. urea.

(iii) By preventing the reabsorption of salts by the renal tubules thereby ensuring an increased excretion especially of sodium. The most effective and important diuretics, e.g. the mercurials, act in this way.

It follows, therefore, that when a diuretic is given to reduce œdema there must also be a restriction of fluid and salt intake.

The drugs used as diuretics may be classified thus:

I. The major diuretics.

    (*a*) Mercurial diuretics, e.g. mersalyl, 'Neptal'.

    (*b*) Non-mercurial diuretics, e.g. acetazolamide ('Diamox'), chlorothiazide ('Saluric'), bendrofluazide hydroflumethazide, chlorthalidone ('Hygroton') etc.

II. The minor diuretics.

    (*a*) The saline diuretics, e.g. potassium citrate.

    (*b*) Urea.

    (*c*) Diuretics of the caffeine group.

    (*d*) Cardiac diuretics, e.g. digitalis.

The major diuretics are the only ones in general use in the treatment of the severe œdema of congestive heart failure and the other conditions mentioned above.

## I. The Major Diuretics

### (a) Mercurial diuretics

The most powerful diuretics belong to this group and on account of their irritating effect on the kidneys are not used in cases of acute nephritis. Their main use is in cardiac œdema, but they are occasionally used with caution in cases of dropsy due to chronic nephritis.

**Mersalyl** (*Mersalylum*, B.P.)

This is the "official" drug of the group and is a complicated organic compound of mercury. Mersalyl may be given by intramuscular injection (*Injectio mersalyli*) 0·5 to 2 ml., 8 to 30 minims. It has been given intravenously diluted with 10 ml.

of normal saline, but this method is dangerous and has caused fatal collapse in some cases.

The action of mersalyl and similar drugs is increased by the previous administration of ammonium chloride, two capsules each containing 0·5 gram two hours before the injection. Two capsules containing the same amount of potassium chloride may also be given at the same time.

Intramuscular injections should be made deeply into the upper and outer quadrant of the gluteus maximus or outer side of the thigh, care being taken that the point of the needle is in the muscle. Local œdema should, if necessary, be dispersed by pressure before the needle is inserted. If very painful, 2 ml. of 1 per cent procaine may be injected through the needle before the mersalyl. Subcutaneous injection is liable to produce sloughing of the tissues.

If not previously used it is customary to give a test dose of 0·5 ml. and if there is no reaction such as a rash, rigor, nausea, vomiting or severe local pain, to inject 2 ml. the following morning in order that diuresis shall not disturb the patient's sleep.

The mercury takes two to three days to be excreted so that, as a rule, not more than two injections are given weekly. After gross œdema has been dispersed it is often possible to maintain the patient on one weekly injection for a prolonged period.

Patients having mercurial diuretics are usually on restricted fluids and a salt-free diet. After a long course of injections, however, sodium chloride deficiency characterised by weakness, vomiting and failure of the drug to produce diuresis may develop. In a prolonged maintenance course, therefore, salt restriction is less severe and salt may be permitted in cooking. An intake and output chart should be kept.

Proprietary drugs of a similar type include 'Neptal', 'Novurit', 'Salyrgan', 'Esidrone' and 'Thiomerin' (mercaptomerin). The latter may be given subcutaneously but causes pain and local swelling in some patients.

### (b) Non-Mercurial diuretics

**Chlorothiazide** ('Saluric'). Dose 0·5-2 grams daily.

This, together with a number of drugs which have a similar basic chemical composition, is a very potent non-mercurial diuretic which is administered by mouth. The effect of 2 grams is equivalent to that of 2 ml. of mersalyl injection. It acts on the renal tubules causing an increased excretion of water, sodium and to a lesser extent of potassium.

It may be given on alternate days or for the first three or four consecutive days in any one week. 1 gram is given between 6 and 8 a.m. and 1 gram between 12 noon and 2 p.m. in order that the main diuresis may occur before the patient goes to sleep. Later these doses may be reduced to 0·5 gram.

In view of the possibility of potassium depletion it is advisable to give 1 gram of potassium chloride daily at the same time when the course of treatment is prolonged.

**Chlorthalidone** ('Hygroton') is less likely to cause potassium loss and only one morning dose on alternate days or twice weekly is necessary.

Chlorothiazide and the allied drugs increase the action of hypotensive drugs so that the dose of these must be reduced if one happens to be used at the same time otherwise an excessive fall in blood pressure may be caused. Sensitivity to the action of digitalis may also be increased.

Acetazolamide ('Diamox') is a less powerful and less reliable oral diuretic which may be of value in maintaining a patient free from œdema after initial treatment with mersalyl or chlorothiazide.

## II. The Minor Diuretics

### (a) *The saline diuretics*

Potassium citrate (4 grams, 15 to 60 grains) which, in addition to turning the urine alkaline, has a mild diuretic effect.

### (b) *Urea*

Urea, which is normally present in the blood and excreted in the urine, acts as a diuretic if additional large doses are given by mouth, e.g. 1 gram (15 grains) in 60 ml. of water, three times daily.

### (c) *Diuretics of the caffeine group*

**Caffeine** (*Caffeina*)

This is an alkaloid which has diuretic properties. In addition it stimulates the nervous system, causing wakefulness and increased mental activity. In medicinal doses it also stimulates the vasomotor centre and the heart-muscle to some extent. It is present in small quantities in coffee which explains the mildly stimulating and diuretic effect of this beverage. Preparations include:

Caffeine (*Caffeina*), 300 mg. (2 to 5 grains).
Caffeine citrate (*Caffeinæ citras*) 0·6 gram (2 to 10 grains).

### (d) Cardiac diuretics

It has already been explained that digitalis acts as a diuretic in heart disease by reason of the improvement of the general circulation which, in turn, increases the blood-supply to the kidneys. It is, of course, of special value in cases of heart failure, with œdema due to atrial fibrillation. It does not increase the urinary output in normal persons.

## Methods of reducing general œdema

One of the causes of generalised œdema is the retention of sodium within the body which, in turn, causes the retention of an excess of fluid in the tissues.

In treating such cases the following methods are employed:

1. Diuretics to increase fluid output by the kidneys.
2. Restricted fluid intake.
3. Restricted sodium intake (salt-free diet).
4. The use of cation exchange resins.

*Cation Exchange Resins* are substances which prevent the absorption of sodium from the alimentary canal and which can, therefore, be used to assist the effects of the other forms of therapy, e.g. 'Katonium', average dose 15 grams twice daily with meals. It is important to check the blood electrolytes during their use as they may cause potassium deficiency.

Other methods of removing surplus fluid from the body include:

Paracentesis thoracis.
Paracentesis abdominis.
Southey's tubes, inserted into œdematous legs.
Incision on the dorsum of the œdematous feet.

## DRUGS RENDERING THE URINE ALKALINE

The urine is normally slightly acid in reaction, i.e. it turns blue litmus red.

In addition to this method of indicating the reaction of urine (or any other liquid), the reaction may also be stated in terms of what is called the hydrogen-ion concentration or $p$H. A solution which is neutral is described as having a $p$H of 7. Acid solutions have a $p$H of less than 7 (e.g. *p*H 5) while alkaline solutions have a *p*H greater than 7 (e.g. *p*H 9). Special indicators are required to determine *p*H accurately.

It is frequently desirable to render the urine alkaline, for example to hinder the growth of organisms, especially the *Bacillus coli*, which does not flourish in alkaline urine. Alkalis are therefore given in cases of pyelitis and cystitis, particularly in the acute stages. Strongly acid urine is also irritating to the bladder and in some cases may cause frequent and painful micturition.

Alkalis, usually given in mixture form, include:

Potassium citrate (*Potassii citras*)  
Sodium citrate (*Sodii citras*)  } 4 grams,  
Sodium bicarbonate (*Sodii bicarbonas*)  } 15 to 60 grains.

## DRUGS RENDERING THE URINE ACID

Drugs are occasionally given to make the urine acid in order to permit the efficient action of other drugs which are only effective in an acid medium. For example, mandelic acid and its preparations are only effective as urinary antiseptics against the *Bacillus coli* in acid urine (*p*H 5·5).

The following salts are used:

Acid sodium phosphate (*Sodii phosphas acidus*), 16 grams, 30 to 240 grains.

Ammonium chloride (*Ammonii chloridum*), 4 grams (5 to 60 grains).

## URINARY ANTISEPTICS

Urinary antiseptics are drugs which, when given by mouth, are excreted by the kidneys and have the power of inhibiting the growth of organisms in the urine. The most important urinary antiseptics are:

Sulphonamides.            Antibiotics.

### The sulphonamides

In addition to their action on streptococcal, pneumococcal, meningococcal and other infections in various parts of the body, drugs of this group are of special value in infections of the urinary tract due to the *Bacillus coli*. They are, therefore, used in the treatment of pyelitis and cystitis. They are also effective against the gonococcus (page 225). Most soluble sulphonamides act as urinary antiseptics. *Sulphamethizole* ('Urolucosil'), 100-200 mg. every four hours, is specially employed for this purpose.

## Antibiotics

Various antibiotics may be used depending on the organism present in the urine and its sensitivity, especially if it is unaffected by sulphonamides. Streptomycin is often useful in special cases, but it must be remembered that *Bacillus coli* is insensitive to penicillin.

### Other Urinary Antiseptics

**Nitrofurantoin** ('Furadantin'), 5-8 mg. per kilo body weight. This substance is active both against Gram-positive and Gram-negative organisms, including staphylococci and *B. proteus*. The average adult dose is 100 mg. three times daily.

#### Mandelic acid

Mandelic acid or one of its preparations acts as a urinary antiseptic when excreted into the urine. It is essential, however, to have a certain degree of acidity present which is measured, not by litmus, but by a special indicator recording the hydrogen-ion concentration or $p$H. This should not exceed 5·5.

Proprietary preparations include: 'Mandelix', 'Mandecal', 'Mandelamine', 'Ammoket'.

**Hexamine** ('Urotropine'), 2 grams (10 to 30 grains). A rarely used urinary antiseptic acting only in acid urine.

### *The treatment of pyelitis* (summary)

Although there are various methods available, the one very commonly employed is to give sodium or potassium citrate in sufficient doses to render the urine alkaline, together with one of the sulphonamide drugs for 5 or 6 days. If it is unsuccessful, one of the other methods may then be tried. It is most important to ascertain the nature of the infecting organism and, if necessary its sensitivity, from a catheter specimen of urine.

## DRUGS ACTING ON THE BLADDER

The alkalis and urinary antiseptics already mentioned are given by mouth in cases of cystitis. Hyoscyamus is often included in alkaline mixtures because it has a sedative action on the bladder and helps to relieve the symptoms of frequent or painful micturition.

Local applications are also used for washing out the bladder, particularly in cases of chronic cystitis and after operations involving the bladder.

2 pints of fluid at a temperature of 110°F. from a douche can 3 feet above the patient are generally employed, e.g.:

Sodium bicarbonate (1 to 2 per cent).

Dilute acetic acid ($\frac{1}{2}$ per cent).

Oxycyanide of mercury (1 in 4000).

Potassium permanganate (1 in 4000).

Silver nitrate (1 in 10,000, increasing to 1 in 2000).

Drugs such as carbachol have an action on the muscle of the bladder causing it to contract and may be useful in the treatment of post-operative retention of urine.

## DRUGS ACTING ON THE URETHRA

The main condition requiring treatment is urethritis, which is usually due to the gonococcus but may be due to other causes.

Sulphonamides or antibiotics are given orally.

Local applications are sometimes employed, e.g. urethral irrigations with potassium permanganate, 1 in 8000.

In order to produce local anæsthesia of the urethra, procaine, 5 per cent, is injected with a special syringe.

## DRUGS USED IN THE DIAGNOSIS OF URINARY CONDITIONS

The efficiency of the kidneys may be investigated by testing their power of excreting various substances.

### (i) Urea

Urea is normally excreted by the kidneys and the urine contains approximately 2 per cent.

*Urea concentration test.* No fluid is taken for several hours, the bladder is then emptied and the patient given 15 grams of urea by mouth dissolved in 100 ml. of water. The urine is collected 1 and 2 hours later. The amount of urea in each specimen is then estimated. If the concentrating power of the kidneys is normal, the first specimen should contain at least 1·5 per cent and the second 2 per cent of urea.

*Urea clearance test.* There are several methods of performing this test, which depends on comparing the blood urea with the output of urea in the urine. The bladder should be completely emptied at 10 a.m., 11 a.m. and 12 noon (accurate collection is essential and a catheter must be used if necessary). The 10 a.m. specimen is rejected. Blood is taken at 11 a.m. for urea estimation and the amount of urea is estimated in the two specimens of urine.

## (ii) Dyes

Various dyes given by intramuscular or intravenous injection are excreted by the kidneys and colour the urine (see page 48).

By passing ureteric catheters after cystoscopy, the urine from each kidney can be collected separately and the time taken for the dye to appear in the urine from each kidney can be estimated. A delay will indicate damage to one or both kidneys.

The dyes used include:

Indigocarmine, intramuscular, 50 to 100 mg.
                intravenous, 8 to 16 mg.
Methylene blue, intramuscular, 1 ml. of 5 per cent solution.

## (iii) Radio-opaque substances

An outline of the urinary tract obtained by X-rays after the introduction of a radio-opaque substance is called a pyelogram. This may be obtained in the following ways.

### (a) Excretion or intravenous pyelography

The intravenous injection of:

Iodoxyl (B.P.) $\begin{cases} \text{'Pyelectan'.} \\ \text{'Uroselectan B'.} \\ \text{'Uropac'.} \end{cases}$
Diodone (B.P.) 'Perabrodil'.

These iodine-containing substances are excreted by the kidneys and, being opaque to X-rays, radiograms taken 10, 30 and 50 minutes after injection show the outline of the pelvis of the kidneys, the ureters and the bladder.

Diodone is sometimes given subcutaneously with hyalase but Iodoxyl is not used in this manner because it is too irritating. When given intravenously care must be taken that none of the fluid escapes from the vein or a painful arm will result.

## (b) *Instrumental or retrograde pyelography*

A cystoscope is passed and the orifices of the ureters in the bladder determined. After a catheter has been introduced into one or both ureters, 5 to 10 ml. of sterile 20 per cent solution of sodium iodide or sodium bromide are injected, the injection ceasing when the patient complains of pain in the loin. The solution is opaque to X-rays and in this way the outline of the pelvis of the kidney is obtained.

### DRUGS ALTERING THE COLOUR OF THE URINE

Normal urine is described as straw-coloured, amber or like pale sherry. The following abnormalities of colour may occur:

Bright yellow: due to santonin in acid urine.

Pink or red: due to rhubarb or senna, also phenolphthalein.

Black or brown: due to bile, poisoning with phenol or lysol.

Blue or green: due to methylene blue.

# CHAPTER 11

# DRUGS ACTING ON THE NERVOUS SYSTEM

The nervous system may be divided into three main portions:

1. The brain and spinal cord or central nervous system.
2. The nerves or peripheral nervous system.
3. The involuntary (sympathetic and autonomic) system.

The functioning elements of the system are different types of nerve-cells and their fibres.

Nerve-cells and fibres are sensitive to the action of various drugs which reach them via the blood and the cerebrospinal fluid. Their activities may either be stimulated, depressed or altered in function by the action of drugs.

## DRUGS WHICH DEPRESS THE CENTRAL NERVOUS SYSTEM

One of the features of a number of drugs, which in full doses have the effect of depressing the nervous system, is that in small doses they often have an apparently stimulating action. This is shown, for example, in the exhilarating effect of small or moderate doses of alcohol and in the excitement stage manifested during the induction of general anæsthesia.

It may be that in small doses such substances do have an initial stimulating effect. However, it must be remembered that the highest centres of the brain, namely those which are concerned with consciousness and behaviour, are the first to be affected and, normally, these centres exercise a restraining influence on the activities of an individual. It is, therefore, much more likely that these drugs exercise their depressing effect from the commencement and that the apparent stimulation is merely the result of removing the controlling action of the higher centres.

As the dosage of such drugs is increased, other centres or levels of nervous activity are depressed. Sensation is dulled, consciousness is lost, the cough and vomiting reflexes are abolished. Finally, in toxic doses, the vital centres such as the respiratory and vasomotor centres are affected, and if these are completely paralysed death ensues.

From the point of view of therapeutics these drugs may be divided into the following groups:

I. *General anæsthetics*, or drugs used to produce loss of consciousness and muscular relaxation sufficient to allow the performance of surgical operations.

II. *Hypnotics* or drugs used to produce sleep or a general dulling of mental activity.

III. *Tranquilizers* or drugs which allay anxiety and nervous tension.

IV. *Thymoleptic* drugs which alter the mood and general outlook of the depressed or disturbed patient.

V. *Analgesics*, or drugs given to dull the sensation of pain. Such drugs may also act as hypnotics, e.g. morphine, which has both hypnotic and analgesic properties.

If used in poisonous doses, both hypnotics and many analgesics may produce loss of consciousness.

## General anæsthetics

Although chloroform, introduced by Simpson in 1847, was the first anæsthetic to come into general use, the anæsthetic properties of nitrous oxide were observed by Davy in 1798, and Long used ether in 1842.

Drugs used in the production of general anæsthesia fall into three main classes:

1. Volatile substances, the vapour of which is inhaled, e.g.

| | |
|---|---|
| Chloroform. | Trichlorethylene ('Trilene'). |
| Ether. | Vinyl ether ('Vinesthene'). |
| Ethyl chloride. | Halothane ('Fluothane'). |

2. Gases, such as:

Nitrous oxide.  Cyclopropane.

3. Substances given by:

Intravenous injection, e.g. Thiopentone sodium, B.P. ('Pentothal').

Rectal injection, e.g. Bromethol, B.P. ('Avertin').

## 1. Volatile substances

During the induction of anæsthesia with volatile anæsthetics the patient passes through three stages, which are best shown during the administration of chloroform. With modern methods and the induction with intravenous thiopentone these are not now observed.

(a) The stage of mental dullness.
(b) The stage of excitement.
(c) The stage of full anæsthesia.

(a) **The stage of mental dullness.** The first effect is a sensation of slight suffocation and warmth of the body due to dilatation of the blood-vessels in the skin. The senses become less acute, voices appear distant and may be replaced by ringing sounds and other noises. The patient has a "far away" feeling and to some extent the appreciation of pain becomes dulled though not necessarily abolished.

(b) **The stage of excitement.** This is variable. In children it is often non-existent; in some, scarcely evident; in others, slight movements may become violent struggles, secrets may become common property, bad language in one person may have its counterpart in prayer in another, abuse may alternate with protestations of affection, while the vocal efforts may be ecclesiastical in character, operatic or reminiscent of the music hall.

(c) **The stage of anæsthesia.** The third stage of complete anæsthesia is ushered in as the muscles relax and the struggles cease. Vocal refrains give place to regular breathing, which tends to become slower and more shallow as the depth of anæsthesia increases. The pupils contract somewhat, only to dilate again if the anæsthesia becomes dangerously deep, the corneal reflex is lost and finally there is no longer any pupillary reaction to light. The cough reflex is abolished and unless the jaw is supported, the tongue tends to fall back and impede respiration.

The pulse generally remains steady in rate and regular in rhythm, unless the patient is gravely ill or the operation is very prolonged, when it may become more rapid, weaker and, sometimes, irregular. Blood-pressure tends to fall a little, except with ether anæsthesia, during which it is generally maintained. In some instances the fall may be considerable and cause grave anxiety.

During recovery, the patient returns to consciousness through the same stages, although they may be less obvious. Reflexes return, there is often some degree of restlessness and, finally, a period of drowsiness and dulled mental state before full recovery is attained.

SUMMARY

(i) Anæsthetics given by inhalation reach the lungs in the inspired air. They pass through the alveoli into the blood, by which they are carried in the red corpuscles to the cells of the brain. Here they act by depressing the activity of the cells to such an extent that consciousness is lost.

(ii) The tendon, pupillary and corneal reflexes are lost.

(iii) The cough and vomiting reflexes are lost.

(iv) The muscles are relaxed.

(v) The blood-pressure falls, especially with chloroform anæsthesia, but is not markedly affected by ether.

(vi) The blood-vessels of the skin are dilated. Therefore, there is a tendency to considerable loss of heat from the body. This is minimized by clothing the patient suitably in a flannel gown and woollen stockings, by hot blankets and by maintaining the temperature of the operating theatre.

(vii) Chloroform has a depressing action on the heart, and if administration is prolonged, the pulse tends to become rapid and weak. Ether is a cardiac stimulant and, therefore, the strength of the pulse tends to be maintained, unless the operation is unduly lengthy or is a severe one associated with a great deal of shock.

(viii) Volatile anæsthetics are excreted from the body mainly by the lungs. Therefore the inhalation of carbon dioxide and oxygen mixture after the administration has ceased stimulates the respiratory centre so that the increased rate and depth of breathing hastens their excretion (page 114).

(ix) Ether, in particular, produces an increase in bronchial secretion, which may be very troublesome. In order to prevent this, a pre-anæsthetic injection of atropine sulphate (0·5 to 1 mg., or $\frac{1}{100}$ grain approx.) is given.

N.B.—There are three important questions which a nurse should ask, and verify, of every patient about to have a general anæsthetic, viz.:

(1) Have you any false teeth?

(2) Have you had any food or drink during the last four hours?

(3) Is the bladder empty?

## Chloroform  (*Chloroformum*)

Chloroform is a heavy volatile liquid having a characteristic sweetish odour. It is a very powerful anæsthetic, which is usually administered in drops on an open mask. It is

occasionally mixed with ether in various proportions, especially for the induction of anæsthesia (e.g. chloroform 2 parts,
ether 3 parts).

It has the following advantages:

(i) The production of smooth anæsthesia with good muscular
relaxation.

(ii) It does not irritate the bronchi.

(iii) It is non-inflammable and therefore can be used in safety in
the presence of the cautery or diathermy apparatus.

The disadvantages are:

(i) It is liable to produce dangerous depression of the respiratory
centre.

(ii) It causes a fall in blood-pressure.

(iii) Fatal syncope due to sudden heart failure may occur during
the early stages of induction. The risk of this fatal complication is
increased if adrenaline has been given, and reduced by the pre-
anæsthetic injection of atropine.

(iv) In some instances it has a toxic effect on the liver which may
prove fatal. The symptoms, which include jaundice and vomiting,
may not be apparent for several days after its administration. This
condition is known as "delayed chloroform poisoning". The treatment is to give glucose and insulin.

In view of the fact that, in the past, chloroform has been
responsible for more anæsthetic deaths than any other drug,
it has fallen into disfavour and is now only used for selected
cases.

**Other uses.** Inhalation is sometimes used to relieve pain in
severe renal and biliary colic. The convulsions of status epilepticus,
uræmia, and hypertensive cerebral attacks are also controlled by
inhalations of small doses.

A weak solution in water (Chloroform water—*Aqua chloroformi*)
is used as a flavouring agent for mixtures.

## Ether

This is a light, colourless, highly volatile liquid which
evaporates very quickly and produces a marked cooling of
the body surface to which it is applied. It dissolves fat and
oil and is sometimes used for cleaning the skin, especially
when an injured area is contaminated with oil or grease. It
undergoes chemical change if exposed to strong light and is
therefore kept in amber-coloured bottles.

It may be administered by the "open method" on a mask
or by a "closed method" using a special anæsthetic apparatus.
The endotracheal (intratracheal) route may also be used.

It has the following advantages as an anæsthetic:

(i) It does not depress the respiratory centre or the heart except in large doses and, therefore, there is a considerable margin of safety in its administration.

(ii) It does not tend to lower the blood-pressure and so is useful in cases of shock.

Disadvantages include:

(i) It tends to irritate the bronchial mucous membrane.

(ii) It is highly inflammable and, when mixed with air or oxygen forms a highly explosive mixture. Under no circumstances must there be a naked light or any apparatus liable to produce a spark, e.g. diathermy; or high temperature, e.g. the electric cautery, in the room while ether is being used.

Metal anæsthetic trolleys and operating tables, etc., with rubber castors are liable to carry a charge of electricity which may produce a small spark, and this has been sufficient to cause explosions and fires, having fatal results. It is therefore customary to "earth" such apparatus by means of a metal chain which makes contact with the ground and to use trolleys with special wheels. "Anti-static" wheels are coloured yellow.

### Ethyl chloride

This is a very volatile liquid which evaporates so rapidly that it produces a freezing effect on the skin. Advantage is taken of this to produce local anæsthesia. It has an unpleasant smell and, for purposes of general anæsthesia, is often mixed with eau de Cologne. Ethyl chloride has a powerful action and induces anæsthesia rapidly. It is only suitable for short operations lasting a few minutes, e.g. tonsillectomy by the guillotine, extraction of teeth, incision of abscesses, etc., and for inducing anæsthesia which is continued by the administration of ether.

It is usually given on an open mask.

### Trichlorethylene ('Trilene')

This is a useful, non-inflammable anæsthetic which is less toxic than chloroform. It is non-irritant to the respiratory passages but does not always produce the complete muscular relaxation necessary for some major operations. It may be used in obstetrics. A blue colour distinguishes it from other liquids.

**Vinyl ether** ('Vinesthene'), 'Neothyl', Halothane.

These are volatile liquids occasionally used.

## 2. *Gaseous substances*

### Nitrous oxide $(N_2O)$

Nitrous oxide is a colourless gas having a very faint odour and sweetish taste. It is the oldest anæsthetic and its early name "laughing gas" is indicative of the hilarity which may be produced during the excitement stage of induction or recovery. It is stored in cylinders and administered via a bag and rubber face-piece, either directly from the cylinders for short anæsthesia, or by means of more elaborate apparatus for prolonged administration.

Nitrous oxide when inhaled for about half a minute produces anæsthesia lasting approximately 40 seconds, which is sufficient for some dental extractions, opening abscesses, etc. During its inhalation, however, the patient is deprived of oxygen and therefore cyanosis develops quickly and, at the same time, muscular spasms (jactitation) are frequently observed.

When nitrous oxide is mixed with oxygen, anæsthesia can be prolonged almost indefinitely without harmful effects. In major surgical procedures it is usual to give a hypnotic such as morphine or 'Omnopon' and scopolamine (hyoscine) beforehand, or a basal anæsthetic (page 144) may be used. It may be necessary to supplement its administration with small doses of ether in order to produce full muscular relaxation.

Advantages:

(i) Given with oxygen it is one of the safest of all anæsthetics.

(ii) It does not lower blood-pressure or increase shock.

(iii) It rarely produces vomiting.

(iv) It may be given by the endotracheal method or nasally.

Disadvantages:
  (i) Cumbersome and expensive apparatus is necessary for its administration,
  (ii) It is not always possible to obtain full muscular relaxation without adequate premedication with a hypnotic or basal anæsthetic, and the addition of ether may be necessary. The quantity of ether required, however, is much less than when ether is used alone and, in this respect, nitrous oxide is one of the most useful anæsthetics available.

**Use in midwifery.** Inhalations of nitrous oxide and air (which in this instance supplies an adequate amount of oxygen) are administered by the patient herself in order to produce analgesia during labour, similar to that obtained by chloroform capsules. A special apparatus, e.g. Minnett's, is required. Valves are so arranged that an overdose is not possible and, in any case, the face-piece will fall from the patient's hand if consciousness is actually lost.

## Cyclopropane

This is a non-irritating gas which has powerful anæsthetic properties. It can be given with large amounts of oxygen, with which it may form an explosive mixture. It is only used with safety by experts, but has advantages which render it especially valuable in thoracic surgery.

### 3. Substances given by injection

#### (A) Substances given by intravenous injection

These drugs, which belong to the barbiturate group (page 148), can be used:
  (i) As general anæsthetics for short operations.
  (ii) For longer operations if repeated doses are given or a continuous drip method employed.
  (iii) For induction of anæsthesia followed by ether or nitrous oxide.
  (iv) As basal anæsthetics.
  (v) To control the spasms of tetanus.

They are all extremely quick in action, the patient passing into unconsciousness in less than 30 seconds if given rapidly.

The effect of a full single dose lasts about 15 minutes. This may be prolonged, as stated above, by repeated injections of smaller doses or by a continuous drip method.

Great care must be taken to maintain an efficient airway. The jaw, which always tends to fall back even before the injection has been completed, must be properly supported until recovery from the anæsthetic is in sight.

The patient must be lying flat during the administration as a fall in blood-pressure is produced and, if the patient were allowed to sit up, e.g. in a dental chair, the lack of blood supply to the brain might be sufficient to produce dangerous symptoms. Twitching of the muscles, which may be violent, is sometimes observed.

The solution is a strong irritant and it is most important that none should get into the tissues surrounding the vein.

The immediate injection of 'Hyalase' in normal saline into the area is helpful.

Accidental injection into an artery is even more serious and may lead to gangrene. It is treated by immediate injection of 10 ml. of 1% procaine into the artery.

### Thiopentone sodium, B.P. ('Pentothal')

0·5 gram is dissolved in 10 ml. of sterile distilled water before injection. About 5 ml. are generally required to induce anæsthesia.

### Sodium Amytal, 'Pernocton', 'Nembutal'

These may all be given by intravenous injection.

Some drugs of this type are also given by mouth to produce sleep before anæsthesia, but unless large doses are used it is generally possible to rouse the patient.

Over-dosage and collapse are treated with injections of bemegride ('Megimide') or nikethamide. Other measures which may be adopted in an emergency during general anæsthesia include:

Artificial respiration and external cardiac massage.
Inhalation of carbon dioxide and oxygen.
Cardiac massage after opening the abdomen.

## (B) *Substances given by rectal injection*

The drugs given by rectal injection and also some of those given intravenously are not, strictly speaking, general anæsthetics. That is to say, major surgical operations cannot often be performed under their influence alone, and it is usually necessary to produce deeper anæsthesia by the added use of ether or nitrous oxide. Drugs of this type are called **basal anæsthetics** or basal narcotics. They have the advantage that unconsciousness can be induced before the patient leaves his bed and he is spared the knowledge of the entrance into the operating theatre and the induction of general anæsthesia, which is so frequently feared.

Other advantages are: a smaller dose of other anæsthetics is needed and the patient usually continues to sleep peacefully for some hours after his return to bed.

The dangers are that respiration may be depressed, and once the dose has been given and absorbed it is slowly excreted so that, should the patient collapse, little can be done to hasten recovery from the anæsthetic.

### Bromethol, B.P. ('Avertin')

A freshly prepared 2·5 per cent solution is given per rectum. The exact dose is calculated from the patient's weight, having regard also for his general condition (i.e. 100 mg. per kilogram body weight).

The required amount of bromethol fluid is measured and is added to distilled water at body heat. The solution is shaken thoroughly. The temperature must not exceed 40°C. (104°F.). Solutions are tested before use by adding 2 drops of a 1 in 1000 solution of congo red to 5 ml. of bromethol solution. A bright orange-red colour should persist. If the solution turns blue it must be discarded.

The solution is run into the rectum with a tube and funnel half an hour before the operation. Morphine or hyoscine should not be administered at the same time.

Bromethol may also be used to control the spasms of tetanus.

### Paraldehyde

This drug, which is described under hypnotics (page 151), is sometimes given in appropriate doses per rectum as a basal anæsthetic. Up to 60 minims per stone body weight is given in saline to make a 10 per cent solution. It is less powerful than Bromethol.

## 4. *Aids to Anæsthesia*

### Muscle Relaxants

(*i*) **Tubocurarine.** Preparations of curare and similar substances, e.g. 'Tubarine', gallamine triethiodide ('Flaxedil'), are given by injection in order to increase muscular relaxation, thus diminishing the amount of general anæsthetic necessary. These drugs act by paralysing the nerve-endings in the muscles (myo-neural junction). The average dose is 5-15 mg. by intravenous injection. Suxamethonium may be used.

Neostigmin (2 mg.) preceded by atropine 1 mg. ($\frac{1}{60}$ gr.) is used as an antidote to overdosage.

(*ii*) **Mephenesin** ('**Myanesin**'), 0·5-1 gram (30-15 ml. of 2% solution by slow intravenous injection). This is a synthetic substance which produces some muscular relaxation. It appears to act on the spinal cord and may also be used in strychnine and barbiturate poisoning.

It is also used as a general muscle relaxant in a number of spastic conditions and may be given by mouth in the form of an elixir. It may be used in sedative preparations given in anxiety states.

## Hypnotics

In some respects it is difficult to divide hypnotics and analgesics into separate groups, for there are a number of the former which have analgesic properties as well. When given in ordinary doses they can be classified as:

1. Drugs having hypnotic effects only.
2. Drugs having analgesic effects only.
3. Drugs having both hypnotic and analgesic affects. The last group consists of individual drugs and preparations made by mixing drugs of the first two types.

### 1. Drugs having hypnotic effects only

A hypnotic or narcotic drug is one which is used to induce sleep and also has a calming or sedative action on the nervous system. It is, in fact, a substance which the lay person regards as a "drug". An analgesic relieves pain. Substances having both actions are therefore used especially to treat insomnia or sleeplessness when the patient is unable to sleep on account of pain. They may also be used to relieve severe pain irrespective of their narcotic effects, e.g. morphine. For minor degrees of pain a simple analgesic, such as aspirin, is usually all that is required.

*Drug addiction.* Great care and discrimination must be exercised in the use of these drugs. Many are "habit-forming";

that is, the patient feels unable to do without them. Others, if given over a period, result in a serious craving for the drug when it is withdrawn. Drug addiction is a very difficult condition to cure and sufferers will often go to extremes in order to obtain the drug and satisfy their cravings. For this reason the sale and issue of most of the drugs of this type is controlled by the Dangerous Drugs Act and they can only be obtained on a doctor's prescription (page 6).

**Insomnia.** The inability to secure sufficient sleep, or failure to obtain sound restful sleep, is a problem which frequently presents itself for treatment, and it is not solved by simply prescribing one of the many available hypnotic drugs.

The first step is to ascertain, if possible, the underlying cause. A simple method of grouping cases is:

1. Primary—where no physical cause can be found, e.g. anxiety states, hysteria.

2. Secondary—where pain, physical discomfort such as indigestion—irritation of the skin (pruritus)—frequency of micturition—cough—or some organic disease, is the cause.

In the second group, treatment is given for the underlying cause and its symptoms before, or at the same time as, active measures are adopted to procure sleep.

*General Management*

A careful history of the patient's habits must be obtained so that any undesirable factors or contributory causes may be eliminated.

1. He should sleep in a quiet room, adequately ventilated but kept at an even temperature. The blinds should be drawn, doors and windows wedged to prevent rattling and clocks removed. (Occasionally the monotonous ticking of a clock is an aid to drowsiness.)

2. The bed-clothes should be light but warm. As a rule, a spring mattress is best, but it is not always wise to change the type of bed to which the patient is accustomed.

3. A warm bath on retiring promotes sleep in some indi-

viduals. A hot-water bottle or bed-socks are often of value, especially if coldness of the extremities is noticed.

4. Overloading the stomach shortly before bed-time is undesirable and a light evening meal is often preferable to a heavy dinner. In such circumstances, soup, Bovril, hot milk or a preparation such as Ovaltine may be taken just before retiring, or during the night if the patient wakes, provided it is kept hot in a Thermos flask and the patient does not have to rouse himself to prepare it.

5. Tea and coffee at night should be avoided. The effect of alcohol is variable. In some patients, whisky or brandy in hot or cold water is of great value as a night-cap while in others it produces wakefulness. Before prescribing it the possibility of producing an alcohol habit must be considered, especially if the patient is of an unbalanced psychological order.

6. Patients who complain of wakefulness on account of excessive mental activity on retiring, should pass their evenings quietly and games such as competitive cards should be avoided. Quiet reading of unsensational literature may be recommended, while the effect of a walk before bed-time may be tried.

7. Many people sleep best on their right side; some prefer one pillow, others like a number, and a few imagine they sleep best with their beds in some definite position, e.g. placed north and south.

8. The patient often fears the consequences of insomnia more than the lack of sleep, a dread which in itself may produce an anxiety state. Reassurance is, therefore, of great importance. He should be told that life will not be lost on this account nor will he lose his reason.

It is clearly wrong to attempt to force the patient to sleep with potent drugs without first attempting to remove the underlying cause. Drugs may be essential in cases of this type in order to obtain the tranquillity of mind necessary for psychotherapy to be effective. They are also valuable in breaking the "habit of insomnia" which is prone to exist in this type of case.

The fact of taking a drug is a powerful suggestive force

which will aid in procuring sleep and, in the first instance, the preparation employed should be strong enough to produce the desired effect. The dose and potency should subsequently be reduced without the knowledge of the patient.

The hypnotic drugs not having any special analgesic action are:

1. The barbiturates.
2. Chloral hydrate and dichloralphenazone ('Welldorm').
3. Paraldehyde.
4. The bromides.
5. Drugs of the urea and sulphone groups.
6. Synthetic drugs such as Glutethimide ('Doriden'), Methyprylone ('Noludar'), which also act as tranquillizers in smaller doses.

## 1. The barbiturates

There are a large number of drugs derived from barbituric acid which have a depressing effect of the central nervous system and are used as hypnotics. They have little effect on pain and are for this reason often combined with analgesic drugs in proprietary preparations.

In addition to their use as hypnotics and general sedatives in anxiety states, certain of them, e.g. phenobarbitone, are employed in the treatment of epilepsy to depress the irritability of the cerebrum.

Although a patient taking barbiturates regularly for insomnia may not be able to sleep properly without them and may come to rely on them, and they are, in this sense, habitforming; they do not tend to produce the craving which may follow the habitual use of drugs like opium, morphine and cocaine.

It is not uncommon to find cases in which an over-dose has been taken either accidentally or with suicidal intent.

Barbiturates should never be used in combination with alcohol or methyl pentynol ('Oblivon') as the drugs have a cumulative effect if taken together. This is most dangerous for car drivers.

The most important barbiturates fall into three main groups, viz.:

1. Short action (3 to 6 hours) rapid excretion, e.g.:

| | | DOSE: mg. | grains |
|---|---|---|---|
| Quinalbarbitone | 'Seconal' | 200 | ¾ to 3 |
| Hexobarbitone | 'Evipan' | 500 | 4 to 8 |
| Cyclobarbitone | 'Phanodorm' | 400 | 3 to 6 |

2. Intermediate action (4 to 8 hours), e.g.:

| | | | |
|---|---|---|---|
| Amylobarbitone | 'Amytal' | 300 | 1½ to 5 |
| Pentobarbitone | 'Nembutal' | 200 | 1 to 3 |
| Butobarbitone | 'Soneryl' | 200 | 1 to 3 |

3. Long acting (8 to 16 hours), e.g.:

| | | | |
|---|---|---|---|
| Phenobarbitone | 'Luminal' | 120 | ½ to 2 |
| Methyl phenobarbitone | 'Prominal' | 200 | 1 to 3 |
| Barbitone sodium | 'Medinal' | 600 | 5 to 10 |

Among the many other drugs containing barbiturates are 'Somnifane', 'Allonal', 'Dial', 'Cibalgin', 'Evidorm'. 'Tuinal' (a mixture of quinalbarbitone and amylobarbitone).

The sodium preparation of the various barbiturates are more soluble than the other forms and act more quickly. Soluble phenobarbitone (sodium) may be given by intramuscular injection (200 mg., 3 grains).

### Symptoms of barbiturate poisoning include:

Increasing coma.

Depression of the respiratory centre with slow, shallow breathing.

Abolition of the tendon and eye reflexes.

Fall in blood-pressure.

Later, bronchopneumonia.

### Treatment of barbiturate poisoning:

1. Gastric aspiration and lavage.
2. Injections of nikethamide.
3. Inhalations of oxygen.
4. Intravenous injection of bemegride ('Megimide'), an analeptic drug having a longer action than nikethamide or picrotoxin. 10 ml. of a 0·5 per cent solution of bemegride is injected into the tube of an intravenous 5 per cent dextrose drip at intervals of approximately

5 minutes. Amiphenazole ('Daptazole'), 15 mg. may be given at the same time.

5. Intravenous injection of amphetamine sulphate, 20 to 50 mg.

6. The use of antibiotics with a view to preventing the development of pneumonia in cases in which coma is prolonged.

7. Severe cases may need a mechanical respirator. Sometimes an 'artificial kidney' may be employed.

Barbiturates should be used with special caution in:

1. Allergic patients (asthma, angio-neurotic œdema).

2. Defective renal or hepatic function.

3. Diabetes.

4. Thyrotoxicosis.

5. Old age.

The tendency to habit formation may be greatly diminished by withholding from the patient the knowledge of the name and dose of the drug he is taking.

2. **Chloral hydrate** (*Chloral hydras*), 0·3 to 2 grams (5 to 30 grains)

This is a drug which occurs in crystalline form but is usually dissolved in water and given in the form of a mixture or draught. It may be combined with a bromide, e.g. *Mistura potassii bromidi et chloralis.*

Chloral hydrate 1·2 gram (20 grains) with 1 ml. (15 minims) of tincture of opium is a useful hypnotic.

Another preparation is syrup of chloral (*Syrupus chloralis*). This is sometimes used for children, but a serious word of warning must be given. Although the official dose of the syrup is up to 8 ml. (30 to 120 minims), this is an adult dose, and 4 ml. (60 minims) contain about 700 mg. (11 grains) of chloral. This is a very large and dangerous dose for a child, even though infants tolerate chloral well. A suitable dose for an infant of 1 year is 120 mg. (2 grains) i.e. not more than 1 ml. (15 minims) of syrup of chloral.

Chloral is a very effective hypnotic which does not predispose to habit formation. It is quite safe to give to cardiac cases in ordinary doses, although at one time this was thought to be inadvisable.

'Welldorm' is a proprietary tablet or elixir containing dichloralphenazone.

**3. Paraldehyde** (*Paraldehydum*), oral dose $\begin{cases} 2 \text{ to } 8 \text{ ml.} \\ 30 \text{ to } 120 \text{ minims.} \end{cases}$

This is a colourless liquid with a characteristic pungent odour and unpleasant taste. It is, however, a very safe and valuable hypnotic. Its duration of action is relatively short and it is excreted in the breath so that it can be smelt some hours after its administration.

Paraldehyde is now usually given by intramuscular injection (*Injectio paraldehydi*, dose, 5 to 10 ml.).

It is sometimes prescribed in mixture form for oral administration, but is only slightly soluble in water. The bottle must be carefully shaken as the bulk of the paraldehyde tends to float on the top of the mixture.

It can also be given per rectum, when double the oral dose may be ordered.

Accidents have sometimes happened, and proved fatal, because the dose of paraldehyde has been misread. It must be emphasized that the dose of pure paraldehyde is measured in minims, drachms or millilitres; and only when previously mixed with water will the dose be ordered as one or more ounces. The nurse must always make quite certain which of the two she is using.

### 4. The bromides

Bromides are crystalline salts which are soluble in water, e.g.

Potassium bromide (*Potassii bromidum*) ⎤
Sodium bromide (*Sodii bromidum*) ⎬ 0·3 to 2 grams
Ammonium bromide (*Ammonii bromidum*) ⎦ 5 to 30 grains.

They are usually given in mixture form and have a general sedative effect on the nervous system. In order to produce sleep they may be given with chloral.

Bromides have largely been replaced by barbiturates in the

treatment of epilepsy and as nerve sedatives in cases of mental anxiety and states of excitement.

"Bromism" (page 29) may develop in persons especially sensitive to bromide (idiosyncrasy) and in cases of over-dosage. The symptoms include skin eruptions which resemble acne or eczema. Bromides are not well tolerated by the elderly and, therefore, should be used with caution in old age, for they are then liable to cause mental confusion. They have no special habit-forming properties.

5. **The urea group** contains some mild and safe hypnotics, e.g.

| | |
|---|---|
| Urethane | 2 grams, 15 to 30 grains. |
| Carbromal ('Adalin') | 5 to 15 grains. |
| Bromural | 5 to 10 grains. |

6. **Methylpentynol** ('Oblivon') is a drug which has a seda-tive effect and is particularly useful in allaying apprehension, nervous tension or excitement. It is given in the form of cap-sules or an elixir, but, being an alcohol, should not be com-bined with barbiturates.

### 2. Tranquillizers

In recent years this term has been introduced to cover a number of drugs which are intended to calm the nervous system in states of anxiety and nervous tension.

Most of the hypnotic drugs given in smaller doses than those needed to produce drowsiness or sleep have a tranquillizing effect. In this sense phenobarbitone, amylobarbitone, bro-mides, drugs of the urea group and methyl pentynol may all be used in this way.

In the same way the drugs which are used specially as tranquillizers will have a hypnotic effect if given in excessive dosage.

The non-barbiturate tranquillizers include:

Meprobamate, 400 mg. (6 grains), which is also obtainable in the proprietary forms 'Equanil', 'Mepavlon' and 'Miltown'.
Pecazine, 25-100 mg. ($\frac{2}{5}$-1$\frac{1}{2}$ grains), e.g. 'Pacatal', 'Covatin'.
Hydroxyzine, 10-25 mg. ($\frac{1}{6}$-$\frac{2}{5}$ grain), e.g. 'Atarax'.
Glutethimide, 250 mg. (4 grains), e.g. 'Doriden'. In double this dose 'Doriden' is used as a hypnotic.

Methyprylone ('Noludar') in doses of 50 to 100 mg. is a sedative. The hypnotic dose for insomnia is 200 to 400 mg. Chlorpromazine, ('Largactil') and promazine ('Sparine') may also be used as tranquilizers.

**Chlorpromazine** ('Largactil'). 70-150 mg. ($1\frac{1}{4}$-$2\frac{1}{2}$ grains) daily in divided doses, or 25-50 mg. by deep intramuscular or intravenous injection. Under certain circumstances these doses may be considerably increased. This is a drug which appears to depress the activity of certain parts of the nervous system without actually acting as a hypnotic. It is an anti-emetic and, therefore, of value in the treatment of excessive vomiting in pregnancy and other conditions. It reduces skin irritation and itching and appears to enhance the effect of some analgesics such as pethidine, hence its use in obstetrics. It may be given by mouth in doses of 75 to 140 mg. daily or by deep intramuscular injection (25 mg.). If given intraven-ously it must be well diluted and is best administered in a saline drip (see also page 66). Toxic effects, including jaundice and agranulocytosis, may follow its use.

**Promazine** ('Sparine'), 25-200 mg., up to four times daily, has a similar action but is unlikely to cause jaundice. Much higher dosage may be used in the treatment of psychiatric patients.

### 3. Drugs having analgesic effects (Anodynes)

The most important drugs of this type are:

**Acetylsalicylic acid** (*Acidum acetylsalicylicum*—**Aspirin**), 0.3-1 gram (5-15 grains).

When given by mouth this drug is of great value in relieving minor degrees of pain and discomfort. It also induces sweating and tends to lower the body temperature, i.e. it is also an antipyretic (page 60). Like sodium salicylate, it is of value in the treatment of rheumatism, chorea, neuralgia, fibrositis and in gout.

It is often given in combination with soluble barbitone ('Medinal') or other barbiturates, which have hypnotic effects, while any associated pain is controlled by aspirin.

Aspirin has a slight local anæsthetic action when applied to

F

mucous membranes and so is useful as a gargle to relieve pain after tonsillectomy 0·6 gram in 30 ml. (10 grains in 1 ounce) of water.

It is given either in tablets, containing 300 mg. (5 grains), or in mixture form.

Calcium aspirin, known also as *Tabella acidi acetylsalicylici solubile*, N.F. and 'Disprin' is more soluble than ordinary aspirin. It is therefore more readily absorbed and acts more quickly. It has less tendency to cause gastric irritation.

Tablets containing aspirin mixed with other drugs are also commonly used, e.g.

Compound aspirin tablet (*Tabella acidi acetysalicylici composita*), Tab. A.P.C., containing approximately aspirin 230 mg. (3½ gr.), phenacetin 160 mg. (2½ gr.), caffeine 30 mg. (½ gr.).

Compound codeine tablet (*Tabella codeinæ composita*), contains approximately aspirin 260 mg. (4 gr.), phenacetin 260 mg. (4 gr.), codeine phosphate 8 mg. (⅛ gr.).

'Veganin' is similar in composition to the latter.

'Anadin' contains aspirin, phenacetin, caffeine and quinine sulphate. There are many analgesic preparations, including 'Paynocil', 'Zactirin', and 'Doloxine' containing aspirin in various forms and with other drugs.

**Aspirin poisoning.** Accidental and suicidal aspirin poisoning are not uncommon. The symptoms include nausea, vomiting, noises in the head, rashes, and a weak, rapid pulse. Large doses cause coma and death.

Treatment: The stomach should be washed out, preferably with 5% sodium bicarbonate solution or an emetic may be given. Stimulants e.g. nikethamide may be required for respiratory failure. Milk or water containing bicarbonate by mouth and intravenous fluids, e.g. saline, Dextran or Hartmann's solution may be needed. An 'artificial kidney' may save severe cases.

Aspirin in ordinary doses sometimes causes gastric bleeding and hæmatemesis.

Other pain relieving drugs include: Dihydrocodeine ('D.F.118'), 'Zactirin'. 'Saridone', paracetamol ('Panadol'). The usual dose is one or two tablets.

## Sodium salicylate (2 grams, 10 to 30 grains)

This drug is used especially in the treatment of rheumatic fever in which it reduces the temperature to normal and relieves the joint pains. Full doses must be given at first and then gradually reduced. It is usual to prescribe an equal quantity of sodium bicarbonate at the same time with a view to reducing toxic effects. The symptoms of overdosage are similar to those produced by aspirin.

## Phenacetin (*Phenacetinum*), 600 mg. (5 to 10 grains).

This is an analgesic drug especially used to relieve headache and minor degrees of pain. It is often combined with aspirin and caffeine and given in tablet form.

Amidopyrine acts as an analgesic and antipyretic, but in some persons who show idiosyncrasy it is liable to produce the dangerous condition known as agranulocytosis, in which the polymorpho-nuclear leucocytes of the blood are markedly diminished by reason of a toxic action on the bone marrow (page 103). The modern tendency, therefore, is to restrict its use.

### 3. *Drugs having both hypnotic and analgesic properties*

There are a number of drugs of this type of which opium and its alkaloid morphine are the most important. Their use is controlled by the Dangerous Drugs Act.

## Opium

Opium is the dried juice of certain poppy heads which are grown mainly in China, India and Persia. It is one of the oldest of drugs and its use was known to the Egyptians, Romans and Greeks. Its activity is due to a number of alkaloids, of which the most important is morphine. Opium contains about 10 per cent of morphine and its important pharmacological actions can be attributed to this alkaloid.

## Morphine, 8 to 20 mg. ($\frac{1}{8}$ to $\frac{1}{3}$ grain).

Morphine acts on the central nervous system, depressing the important centres and has a special effect on the sensory nerve cells, which explains its value in the relief of pain.

(a) **Action on the higher centres.** In some persons there is at first a period of well-being or excitement after its administration due to the removal of the control of the highest centres of nervous activity (cf. anæsthetics). This is soon followed by a general dulling of perception so that the patient assumes a drowsy state with diminished power of attention. While this is going on the sensory centres are depressed and the appreciation of pain and discomfort are markedly diminished. Movements tend to become clumsy and the patient passes into a sleep from which, however, he can be easily roused but which returns when he is left undisturbed.

(b) **Action on the medulla.** The *respiratory centre* is depressed so that respiration becomes slower and shallower. A most important action of morphine. It is helpful in the treatment of dyspnœa in cases of left ventricular heart failure with pulmonary œdema.

The *cough reflex centre* is depressed and this makes opium and morphine of value in allaying irritating and useless cough.

The *vomiting centre* is affected in some persons. In such a case, small doses of morphine appear to have a contradictory action and the centre is stimulated so that the patient vomits. In larger doses the centre is depressed by morphine.

The *vasomotor centre* is somewhat depressed, but to a relatively less extent than the respiratory centre.

*Eye reflexes:* The pupils are contracted.

(c) **Action on the alimentary system.** The nerve plexuses in the walls of the bowel are depressed by the action of opium and morphine. This slows down peristalsis, so that constipation results and the fæces tend to become hard and dry from their prolonged stay in the gut, during which additional water is absorbed by the colon. Advantage is taken of this constipating effect in the treatment of some cases of diarrhœa, e.g. kaolin and morphine mixture.

**Morphine poisoning.** The depth of sleep and other effects produced are dependent on the dose of morphine or opium given. The description so far given would apply to the ordinary therapeutic doses, e.g. not exceeding 20 mg. ($\frac{1}{3}$ grain) of morphine. In larger, and therefore, poisonous doses, sleep develops into coma from which it is very difficult to rouse the patient. Reflexes are lost. The depression of the respiratory centre is so marked that the rate of breathing may be slowed to less than 12 per minute. The contracted pupil becomes pin-point in size. The pulse is weak.

*Treatment of morphine poisoning.* The general principle is to stimulate the patient in every way. Also, the stomach should be washed out with a solution of potassium permanganate, 4 grams (60 grains) in 2 gallons of water, even if the drug has been given by injection, as it is probable that some of the drug given in this way is excreted into the stomach. This may be followed by giving strong black coffee. Sometimes gastric aspiration followed by lavage with not more than 1 litre of water is preferred.

If possible, the patient should be kept awake by walking him about, flicking with wet towels, electrical stimulation, etc. If respiration has ceased, artificial respiration must be performed. In other cases, inhalations of carbon dioxide and oxygen are necessary. Injections of nikethamide, strychnine or caffeine are given to stimulate the respiratory centre, and injections of atropine are helpful.

The antidote to morphine poisoning which should always be used is nalorphine ('Lethidrone'), a powerful stimulant of the respiratory centre, which is given in 10 mg. doses intravenously. It may also be used in over-dosage with pethidine and methadone ('Physeptone'). Amiphenazole ('Daptazole') is also used.

**Idiosyncrasy.** Children do not tolerate morphine or opium well, and doses very small in proportion to the age should be given. This is especially important in infants.

It has been pointed out that some individuals tend to show a degree of restlessness after the injection of morphine. In others, vomiting may be severe.

**Tolerance.** The continued use of morphine leads to a fairly rapidly developing tolerance for the drug and larger and larger doses are required in order to produce effective results. This is probably due to the fact that the tissues acquire the ability of destroying morphine more quickly. It is, therefore, not uncommon to find cases (e.g. those suffering from inoperable carcinoma) receiving two or more grains, several times a day. This amount has been reached by increasing the dose gradually over a period of weeks or months. A dose of this size given to an individual unaccustomed to the drug would, of course, have very serious or fatal results.

## Undesirable effects of morphine

1. *On the alimentary system.* Vomiting and constipation have already been mentioned.

2. *On the respiratory system.* Although useful in allaying cough, the fact that morphine depresses the respiratory centre necessitates great care in its employment in cases of respiratory disease, such as pneumonia (later stages), bronchitis and bronchial asthma. It should never be used in the treatment of an asthmatic attack since it can produce fatal results.

3. *Psychological effects.* Morphine is one of the most important substances responsible for drug addiction. While in the Western Hemisphere the habit of opium smoking is rare, it has not been entirely stamped out in the East in spite of recent attempts to control the evil. This habit ultimately renders the addict a nervous wreck, weak in character, with little moral sense and poor in physique.

The craving for the drug is most commonly produced in the West by its prolonged administration during a painful illness. It is, therefore, most important that it should only be used for limited periods in acute disease. Only in conditions such as inoperable carcinoma, which are likely to prove rapidly fatal, is its use justifiable in chronic disease.

The treatment of drug addiction is extremely difficult. The patient must be confined to a special institution, where attempts are made to substitute the offending drug with others in gradually decreasing doses until both have been entirely withdrawn. Relapses after treatment are common.

**Legal control of morphine** (see page 6).

### Preparations of opium

Ipecacuanha and opium powder (*Pulvis ipecacuanhæ et opii*—Dover's powder), 600 mg. (5 to 10 grains).

Tincture of opium (*Tinctura opii*—laudanum), 2 ml. (5 to 30 minims).

'Nepenthe' is a proprietary preparation resembling, but more pleasant to take than tincture of opium. Dose, 2·5 ml. (20 to 40 minims).

Gall and opium ointment (*Unguentum gallæ cum opio*), used in the treatment of hæmorrhoids.

### Preparations of morphine

Morphine sulphate injection (B.P.), 8 to 20 mg. ($\frac{1}{8}$ to $\frac{1}{3}$ grain). Ampoules containing 10·8 mg. ($\frac{1}{6}$ gr.), 16·2 mg. ($\frac{1}{4}$ gr.), 21·6 mg. ($\frac{1}{3}$ gr.) and 32·5 mg. ($\frac{1}{2}$ gr.) are available.

Morphine and atropine injection (B.P.C.). Ampoules of 1 ml. contain approximately 10 mg. ($\frac{1}{6}$ gr.) of morphine and atropine 0·6 mg. ($\frac{1}{100}$ gr.).

Morphine and hyoscine injection. Ampoules of 1 ml. contain morphine 12·2 mg. ($\frac{1}{6}$ gr.) and hyoscine 0·5 mg. ($\frac{1}{100}$ gr.) approx.

Solution of morphine hydrochloride 1 per cent (*Liquor morphinæ hydrochloridi*), 2 ml. (5 to 30 minims).

Morphine suppository (*Suppositorium morphinæ*), contains 15 mg. ($\frac{1}{4}$ grain).

Morphine is generally given by hypodermic injection, but can be given by mouth.

### Drugs resembling morphine

**Papaveretum injection.** Dose, 10-20 mg. ($\frac{1}{6}$ to $\frac{1}{3}$ grain). This contains alkaloids of opium and is the basis of proprietary preparations such as 'Omnopon'.

It has the analgesic and narcotic properties of morphine but produces fewer side-effects.

**Papaverine** (*Papaverina*), (250 mg.) 2 to 4 grains. This also is an alkaloid of opium, which has an antispasmodic action but little analgesic effect. Eupaverine is a similar synthetic substance which is stated to be less toxic. These two drugs must not be confused with Papaveretum, and it will be noted that the doses are different.

'Dromoran' (levorphanol), 1·5 mg., is a proprietary preparation having a similar action to morphine.

**Pethidine** ('Dolantin') D.D.A.

This is a synthetic drug which has an analgesic effect and, although less powerful, may be used instead of morphine in some cases. It is very useful in obstetrics. Its duration of action is rather short and it may be necessary to administer it every three hours. Barbiturates or promazine may be given at the same time. The dose is 25-100 milligrams, either by mouth or subcutaneous injection.

The intravenous dose is 25-50 mg.

Addiction is rapidly acquired, and it may produce dizziness, nausea and sweating.

'Pethilorfan' contains pethidine, 100 mg. with levallorphan, 1·25 mg. in 2 ml. ampoules. The latter drug antagonizes the depressing effect of pethidine on the respiratory centre.

**Methadone** ('Physeptone', 'Amidone'), 5 to 10 mg., D.D.A.

This is a powerful synthetic analgesic having no sedative or hypnotic effect which may be given either by mouth, subcutaneous or intramuscular injection. It may produce minor toxic effects such as nausea, vomiting, dizziness and sweating. These are more likely to occur in ambulant patients, so that patients should remain in bed after it has been given. It is also the basis of a useful cough linctus which usually contains 2 mg. of methadone in 4 ml (60 minims). Children tolerate only very small doses and the linctus should be kept out of their reach.

**Diamorphine (Heroin)**, 5-10 mg., $\frac{1}{24}$ to $\frac{1}{8}$ grain (**D.D.A.**)

This is a drug having a similar action to morphine and is even more likely to produce addiction Its manufacture is therefore forbidden in some countries. It may be given as an injection for the relief of pain and as a sedative. It is also used in a linctus for the relief of troublesome coughs, e.g.

Diamorphine (Heroin) linctus (*Linctus diamorphinæ*), 2 to 8 ml. (30 to 120 minims).

**Codeine** (*Codeina*), 10-60 mg. ($\frac{1}{6}$ to 1 grain).

This is an alkaloid derived from opium, having little tendency to promote habit formation. It has mild analgesic and hypnotic properties and depresses the cough reflex. It may be used for the latter purpose in the form of a linctus:

Codeine linctus (*Linctus codeinæ*), 4 ml. (30 to 60 minims).

It is also included in 'Veganin' tablets (*Tabella Codeinæ composita*) for its analgesic and hypnotic effects.

Dihydrocodeine bitartrate ('D.F.118') is a preparation which has powerful analgesic with only mild hypnotic properties.

**Cannabis** (Indian hemp or *Cannabis indica*) D.D.A.

This is the basis of hashish, the smoking of which is one of the forms of drug addiction. It is rarely used for therapeutic purposes. The following is a description of its action (Cushny) which is included here as an illustration of the effects of certain substances of this type on the drug addict.

"Soon after its administration, the patient passes into a dreamy, semi-conscious state, in which the judgement seems to be lost, while the imagination is untrammelled by its usual restraints. The dreams assume the vividness of visions, are of boundless extravagance, and, of course, vary with the character and pursuits of the individual. In the eastern races they seem generally to partake of an amorous nature. The 'true believer' sees the gardens of paradise and finds himself surrounded by troops of houris of unspeakable beauty, while the less imaginative European finds himself unaccountably happy and feels constrained to active movement, often of a purposeless and even absurd character. Ideas flash through the mind without apparent continuity, and all measurement of time and space is lost."

**Hyoscine** also acts as a hypnotic and sedative (see page 179).

# DRUGS WHICH STIMULATE THE NERVOUS SYSTEM

It has already been mentioned that certain drugs stimulate the respiratory and vasomotor centres in the medulla (e.g. nikethamide, leptazol, strychnine, caffeine). Strychnine and caffeine also have a stimulating effect on other parts of the nervous system and must be considered further. Cocaine also has a stimulating effect.

**Strychnine** (*Strychnina*), 2-8 mg. ($\frac{1}{30}$ to $\frac{1}{8}$ grain).

This is the alkaloid of nux vomica and was used as a constituent of some arrow poisons. The main points about its action are: (1) The highest centres of the brain are not markedly affected by therapeutic doses, although possibly the senses do become more acute after its administration.

(2) Its action in stimulating the respiratory and vasomotor centres has been noted (page 113) but it is now rarely used.

(3) It stimulates the spinal cord so that reflexes are increased and become brisker.

(4) Both strychnine and nux vomica are very bitter and act as "bitters" which improve the appetite and increase the tone of the stomach. They are used as "tonics".

**Strychnine poisoning.** The main symptom is the occurrence of muscular spasms which, with larger doses, become generalized convulsions. They are due to stimulation of the spinal cord and resemble those occurring in tetanus. Consciousness remains unclouded.

Treatment: (*a*) Gastric lavage.

(*b*) Intravenous injection of thiopentone to control convulsions.

(*c*) Barbiturate drugs by mouth.

### Preparations of nux vomica and strychnine

Tincture of nux vomica (*Tinctura nucis vomicæ*), 2 ml. (10 to 30 minims).

Injection of strychnine hydrochloride (*Injectio strychninæ hydrochloridi*), 1 ml. ampoules contain 4 mg. of strychnine ($\frac{1}{16}$ grain in 15 minims).

**Caffeine** (*Caffeina*), 300 mg. (2 to 5 grains).

This drug has a number of actions:

(1) Diuretic (page 126).

(2) Respiratory stimulant (page 113).

(3) Central nervous system stimulant. Caffeine excites the higher centres of the cerebrum, increasing mental activity and sensory impressions. It is often combined with aspirin and phenacetin (A.P.C. tablets).

**Cocaine** (*Cocaina*), 16 mg. ($\frac{1}{8}$ to $\frac{1}{4}$ grain) D.D.A.

This drug has two important and opposite actions when used therapeutically. It stimulates the higher centres of the brain but depresses or paralyses the sensory endings of the peripheral nerves when applied locally (i.e. it acts as a local anæsthetic) (page 164). The former action outweighs much of its value as a local anæsthetic and cocaine itself is only used occasionally. There are, however, many substitutes specially prepared so that the effects on the higher centres are less marked.

*Action on the higher centres.* Cocaine stimulates the mental processes, producing hilarity and loquacity. In larger doses, it results in depression and finally coma. It is very prone to cause drug addiction and gives rise to serious results, with rapid mental and moral deterioration. For this reason its supply is most carefully guarded by the Dangerous Drugs Act.

**Amphetamine sulphate** ('Benzedrine'), 2·5 to 10 mg. ($\frac{1}{24}$ to $\frac{1}{6}$ grain).

The following drugs have a similar action and uses:
Dexamphetamine ('Dexedrine').
Methyl amphetamine ('Methedrine').
These synthetic drugs stimulate the higher centres, produce increased mental alertness and temporarily abolish fatigue. They are useful in certain states of mental depression. Care should be taken not to give them near bed-time as they may result in insomnia. Locally they also have an effect on the nasal mucous membrane like adrenaline and ephedrine (i.e. they are vaso-constrictors) and, when inhaled, are sometimes used for nasal catarrh, hay fever, etc.

They are also useful in narcolepsy, epilepsy, post-alcoholic "hangover" and obesity because in the latter they decrease appetite. Some behaviour disorders of children are benefited. Amphetamine may be given intravenously in barbiturate poisoning. Methylamphetamine when given by intravenous or intramuscular injection (10 to 30 mg.) raises the blood pressure and may be given in cases of shock or collapse.

## Local anæsthetics

Local anæsthetics are drugs which paralyse the sensory nerves in the region of their application, so that the passage of painful stimuli towards the spinal cord becomes impossible.

Motor nerves in the vicinity are also affected. They may be used in the following ways:

1. Direct local applications to mucous membranes, e.g. cocaine.

2. By injection, the same drugs being used for all the following:

(*a*) Injection into the skin and tissues at the site of the operation.

(*b*) Injection around nerves at some distance from the site of the operation so that the area which they supply is anæsthetized, i.e. "regional anæsthesia" produced by nerve-block.

(*c*) "Splanchnic nerve-block", i.e. injection of the nerve ganglia on the posterior abdominal wall which receive the nervous impulses from the abdominal viscera such as the stomach and gall-bladder. This is combined with local anæsthesia of the abdominal wall for some operations.

3. Freezing the skin with ethyl chloride spray.

The ideal requirements of a local anæsthetic are:

1. To paralyse the sensory nerves without damaging them or the surrounding tissues.

2. To be easily sterilized.

3. To be devoid of toxic effects after absorption.

4. To produce anæsthesia of sufficient duration for the operation to be performed and to leave no after-effects.

## I. *Local applications to mucous membranes*

Because of the thinness of the epithelium of mucous membranes, some drugs are absorbed and can easily reach and paralyse the sensory nerve-endings in the vicinity.

(a) **Cocaine,** which is used as a solution (5 to 10 per cent) or ointment (4 to 10 per cent), especially in operations on the nose. The dangers of excessive absorption with toxic symptoms must always be remembered when cocaine is being used. (See also page 162.) Cocaine drops (2 per cent) are of great value in anæsthetizing the conjunctiva prior to the removal of foreign bodies and eye operations. It also dilates the pupil. Solutions of these strengths must never be injected.

(b) **Amethocaine** ('Decicain', 'Pantocaine'), 1 to 2 per cent. This may be used in the same way as cocaine. It is also employed as a spray to anæsthetize the pharynx and larynx before the passage of a gastroscope. It is less toxic than cocaine and, therefore, safer to use but is also considerably more toxic than procaine.

(c) **Benzocaine** ('Anæsthesin') has a similar action and is employed as an injection, lozenge or ointment, viz.:

*Injectio benzocainæ composita* (3%), dose 5 to 10 ml.
*Trochisci benzocainæ compositi.*
*Unguentum benzocainæ compositum.*

## II. Drugs given by injection

These may be injected locally into the operation area (infiltration) or in the vicinity of the nerves which supply the area at some distance from the site of the operation (nerve-block). The most important are:

**Procaine** ('Novocain' or 'Planocaine'). A solution having a strength of ½ to 2 per cent is generally employed. A few drops of 1 in 1000 adrenaline are frequently added. This acts on the blood-vessels in the vicinity of the injection and constricts them, thereby diminishing the amount of procaine which can be carried away in the blood-stream so that the duration of the anæsthesia is prolonged. In addition, the amount of bleeding is diminished. It is occasionally given intravenously for special purposes (0·1 per cent solution).

**Lignocaine** ('Xylocaine') is a local anæsthetic of low toxicity injected as a 0·5 to 2 per cent solution. It is a very stable substance which can be stored indefinitely and repeatedly sterilized in an autoclave.

**Cinchocaine** ('Nupercaine') formerly known as 'Percaine', which is also used as a spinal anæsthetic, must not be confused with procaine. It may be used locally but is very much stronger and more toxic than procaine and, therefore, weaker solutions are employed. It is also made in the form of an ointment.

## III. Freezing the skin

Ethyl chloride spray is sometimes employed and, by its rapid evaporation, freezes the area to which it is applied. The duration of the effect is very short and it is only suitable for incising superficial abscesses. Complete anæsthesia is not always obtained and the process of thawing may be painful.

A *most important warning* must be given in connection with the use of all local and spinal anæsthetics. The names of the substances employed are often similar and may be confused. Further, they are used in strengths varying from 0·5 per cent to 10 per cent. Fatal accidents have occurred from the substitution of 'Percaine' for procaine (hence the advantage of the name 'Nupercaine' or better still, cinchocaine for the former). Also mistakes can be made in reading the strengths on the labels by not observing the exact position of the decimal point. The nurse must therefore be most careful in handling these drugs and be quite sure that the one she is putting out for use is the correct one and in the strength in which it is ordered.

# DRUGS ACTING ON THE PERIPHERAL NERVES AND SPINAL CORD

## Spinal anaesthetics

A number of substances are used for producing spinal anæsthesia. They are introduced by means of lumbar puncture into the subarachnoid space of the spinal canal, where they diffuse in the cerebrospinal fluid and, therefore, surround the spinal cord and the nerve-roots emerging from it in the neighbourhood of the injection. Here they act as local anæsthetics, paralysing the nervous tissue in the nerve-roots so that impulses, both sensory and motor, are unable to pass. It follows that the motor impulses will not be able to pass from the anterior horn cells via the anterior nerve-roots to the muscles which are, therefore, paralysed and completely relaxed. Likewise, sensory impulses coming from the periphery will not be able to enter the cord via the posterior nerve-roots and pass up the sensory tracts to the brain.

The paralysis also involves the nerves to the blood-vessels of the limbs and abdominal organs which dilate and so accommodate more blood. There is thus less blood in the general circulation and the blood-pressure tends to fall.

In order to counteract this effect, it is usual to inject ephedrine (which is a vaso-constrictor) before a spinal anæsthetic is given. In this way, dangerous lowering of the blood-pressure is prevented.

One of the most serious consequences of a fall in blood-pressure is lack of blood to the brain. Lowering of the head of the operating table, an appropriate time after the spinal anæsthetic has been given, counteracts this effect of a fall in blood-pressure.

Spinal anæsthetics are made up in solutions which may be either:

(a) heavier than the cerebrospinal fluid.
(b) lighter than the cerebrospinal fluid.

If the body is tilted so that the head is higher than the feet during the injection, light spinal anæsthetics will tend to rise towards the medulla oblongata. If they reached this level of the spinal cord they would produce respiratory paralysis.

Likewise, if the feet are higher than the head when a heavy spinal anæsthetic is used this will also gravitate towards the medulla. It is, therefore, most important that the appropriate position is maintained by the patient during the injection of all spinal anæsthetics. After a few minutes, however, the anæsthetic becomes "fixed" by the tissues and is no longer free in the spinal canal, so that the patient can be moved into the desired position for the operation, irrespective of the type of drug used.

If there are any signs of collapse during the operation, the head should be lowered in order to increase the blood-supply to the brain, and stimulants such as nikethamide or pholedrine injected.

The most important spinal anæsthetics are:

Cinchocaine ('Nupercaine') (light), 1 in 1500, dose up to 20 ml., (heavy), 1 in 200, dose up to 2 ml.

Amylocaine ('Stovaine') (light and heavy), 1 ml.

Procaine ('Novocain', 'Planocaine', 5 to 10%), 1 to 2 ml.

## Toxic substances acting on nerves

Lead, arsenic, mercury and alcohol may all have an action on the peripheral nerves resulting in peripheral neuritis. Various forms of paralysis ensue. The toxins of the diphtheria bacillus also have a special affinity for nervous tissue.

SUMMARY OF DRUGS USED IN THE TREATMENT OF CERTAIN DISEASES OF THE NERVOUS SYSTEM

## Epilepsy

While it is not possible to state the cause of epilepsy it is clear that the seizures are associated with some local increase in the irritability of the cerebral cortex and that by reducing this irritability by means of anticonvulsant drugs which have a sedative action on the cortex, the fits are controlled or even abolished. The drugs used may be given either alone or two may be combined.

*Phenobarbitone* ('Luminal') 30-120 mg. ($\frac{1}{2}$ to 2 grains) (page 148).

*Phemitone* methylphenobarbitone ('Prominal'). A drug similar in action to phenobarbitone which is said to produce less drowsiness and mental depression.

*Phenytoin* ('Epanutin', 'Solantoin', 'Dilantin', soluble phenytoin) 50-100 mg. is used in some cases which do not respond well to phenobarbitone. Toxic symptoms often occur and include tremor, unsteadiness of movement, swelling of gums, rashes and indigestion.

**Methoin** ('Mesontoin'), 50-100 mg., $\frac{3}{4}$ to $1\frac{1}{2}$ grains.

**Primidone** ('Mysoline'), 250-500 mg..

*Troxidone* ('Tridione', 'Trimethadione'), 1-2 grams, 15 to 30 grains daily in divided doses is specially valuable in *petit mal*. Cases of agranulocytosis have followed its use. 'Paradione' and 'Malidone' are also used for *petit mal*.

*Bromides.* The bromides of potassium, sodium or ammonium are occasionally used 0·6-2 grams (10 to 30 grains). For status epilepticus intramuscular injections of

(*a*) soluble phenobarbitone, 200 mg. (3 grains) or

(*b*) paraldehyde, 5 ml. may be given.

**Syphilis of the nervous system.** The usual antisyphilitic measures are employed (page 212).

**Meningitis.** Sulphonamide drugs are used for meningococcal, streptococcal and pneumococcal types (page 225). Antibiotics may also be required.

**Migraine.** Analgesic drugs such as aspirin, phenacetin or 'Veganin' are given. Ergotamine tartrate ('Femergin') is also used (page 176). Phenobarbitone is of value between attacks.

**Subacute combined degeneration of the cord.** Vitamin $B_{12}$ or liver therapy is necessary (page 100).

**Myasthenia gravis.** Neostigmine (page 177).

**Chorea.** Aspirin or sodium salicylate are given.

**Paralysis agitans** (Parkinsonism). Hyoscine (page 179) or tincture of stramonium (page 119) are given in increasing doses. Pilocarpine 6 mg. ($\frac{1}{10}$ grain) may be necessary to prevent dryness of the mouth. Drugs such as 'Artane', 'Lysivane', 'Pipanol', 'Parpanit', and 'Kemadrin' are also used. Anti-histamines are sometimes helpful.

# CHAPTER 12

# DRUGS ACTING ON THE INVOLUNTARY NERVOUS SYSTEM

It will be recalled that the involuntary nervous system consists of the sympathetic system together with the cranial and sacral autonomic systems (parasympathetic), viz.:

Sympathetic system supplies
- Pupils
- Heart
- Lungs, trachea, bronchi
- Stomach and intestines
- Suprarenal glands
- Bladder
- Uterus

Cranial autonomic supplies
- Pupils
- Heart
- Lungs, trachea, bronchi
- Stomach

Sacral autonomic supplies
- Rectum
- Bladder
- Uterus

The nerve-fibres pass mainly to involuntary, unstriped muscle in the walls of the various organs and also to the muscle in the walls of the arteries, i.e. the autonomic system supplies the viscera as distinct from the central nervous system which supplies the skeletal muscles.

A number of organs have both sympathetic and parasympathetic nerve-supplies which have an antagonistic action towards each other. Thus, the parasympathetic fibres which reach the heart carry impulses which slow the heart-rate (inhibitors), while those from the sympathetic increase its rate (accelerators). The normal rate of the heart is maintained by a balance between the opposing impulses.

Further, the involuntary system is greatly influenced by the activities of the ductless glands. In particular the secretion from the suprarenal gland, adrenaline, stimulates the sympathetic system and acts as a vaso-constrictor.

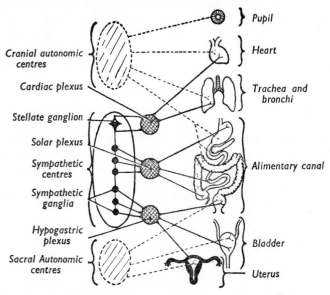

FIG. 5.—Illustrating distribution of Involuntary Nervous System.

Just as reflex action in the central nervous system takes place in the spinal cord, which receives afferent impulses and sends out efferent impulses, so reflex action occurs in the autonomic system through collections of nerve cells called ganglia. These ganglia also have connections with the spinal cord and brain. The sympathetic ganglia are situated in chains on either side of the vertebral column. The parasympathetic ganglia tend to be in or near the organ which they supply and are mainly grouped in the cranial and sacral autonomic centres.

*Physiology.* When an autonomic nerve is stimulated chemical substances are liberated which transmit the impulse at the nerve endings in the organ concerned. Other substances are also formed at the same time which antagonize the action of these stimulators and so prevent their effect being too powerful or too prolonged. These various substances differ in the sympathetic and parasympathetic nerve endings.

Parasympathetic stimulation liberates acetylcholine at the nerve endings. This is antagonized by cholinesterase.

Sympathetic stimulation liberates noradrenaline and adrenaline in addition to acetylcholine. At the same time adrenaline and noradrenaline may be secreted from the suprarenal glands.

Amine oxidase antagonizes their action.

The involuntary system is somewhat complicated and classification of the drugs which affect it is made more difficult by the fact that they all differ in their mode of action. As a matter of convenience they may be divided into three main groups:

1. Those which produce results similar to stimulation of the sympathetic. (sympathomimetic).

2. Those which produce results similar to stimulation of the parasympathetic. (parasympathomimetic).

3. The drugs of the atropine group. (acetylcholine inhibitors).

Drugs acting on the involuntary nervous system may do so in a number of ways. Among the most important are:

1. General stimulants.

2. Ganglion blocking agents which prevent reflex action taking place.

3. Drugs suppressing the action of

   (a) Cholinesterase thus increasing the action of acetylcholine.

   (b) Amine oxidase thus increasing the action of adrenaline and noradrenaline.

4. Drugs inhibiting the action of acetylcholine.

SUMMARY

| Organ | Effect of sympathetic stimulation (adrenaline) | Effect of parasympathetic stimulation (carbachol pilocarpine: eserine) | Action of Atropine |
|---|---|---|---|
| Pupils . . . | Dilated | Contracted | Dilated |
| Heart-rate . . | Increased | Decreased | Increased |
| Bronchial muscle . | Relaxed | Contracted | Relaxed |
| Stomach movements and secretion . | Decreased | Increased | Decreased |
| Saliva . . . | Slight increase | Increased | Decreased |
| Bladder muscle . | Relaxed | Contracted | Relaxed |
| ,, sphincter . | Contracted | Relaxed | — |
| Blood-vessels . . | Contracted | Nil | Nil |

# DRUGS ACTING LIKE SYMPATHETIC STIMULANTS

## Adrenaline

Adrenaline or epinephrine is the active principle extracted from the medulla of the suprarenal glands, and, therefore, normally small amounts are continually passing from the glands into the blood-stream. It is produced synthetically for therapeutic purposes.

If it is remembered that adrenaline stimulates the sympathetic system and that the symptoms of sympathetic stimulation are those which occur in fight or fright, i.e. those actions which are most necessary to the individual for self-preservation, it will not be difficult to understand some of its actions. Thus:

(i) The maximum amount of blood is required for the muscles of the body, therefore there is vaso-constriction of the blood-vessels in the skin and alimentary organs. This also leads to a rise in blood-pressure.

(ii) Glucose is needed in order to supply energy to the muscles, and so the liver liberates its store of glycogen into the blood.

(iii) The plain muscle of the bronchi is relaxed, thus allowing the maximum amount of air to enter the lungs.

*Uses.* (i) Relaxation of the spasm of the bronchial muscles in asthma (see page 119). Small doses of adrenaline (3 to 5 minims, 0·3 ml. of a 1 in 1000 solution, which is the strength in which adrenaline is generally used) are injected immediately the attack starts and are more efficacious than larger ones given when it is fully established. If the responsibility of administering the drug is left to the nurse, she should, therefore, give it as soon as possible. It is not uncommon to be summoned to a patient who has had an attack of asthma which has been in progress for a considerable period, for whom an injection of adrenaline has been ordered "p.r.n." and which could have been given by the nurse at its onset. An intelligent patient may be taught to give the injection to himself.

(ii) As a cardiac stimulant. By constricting the peripheral arteries and those of the abdominal organs the blood-pressure is raised, so that adrenaline is sometimes used in the treatment of shock and collapse. The injection of adrenaline directly into the heart-muscle will sometimes re-start the heart beating when it has stopped, e.g. during anæsthesia, asphyxia, drowning or carbon monoxide poisoning.

(iii) Adrenaline has a powerful local action in constricting the blood-vessels when injected or applied to an open surface, i.e. it is a local hæmostatic. Thus, it may be used as a spray or on gauze soaked in the solution for epistaxis, and for plugging a bleeding tooth socket (see page 58). Its value in delaying the absorption and so prolonging the action of a local anæsthetic has also been mentioned (page 165).

(iv) It is sometimes used in allergic skin conditions such as urticaria, angio-neurotic œdema, hay fever and in anaphylaxis.

Adrenaline is destroyed by the digestive juices and so is inactive when given by mouth.

## Preparations

Injection of adrenaline tartrate (*injectio adrenalini*, B.P.) is issued in ampoules of 0·5 ml. and 1·0 ml. The dose is 2 to 8 minims, i.e. up to ½ ml. Doses of 1 ml. are, however, sometimes given.

Solution of adrenaline hydrochloride (*Liquor adrenalinæ hydrochloridi*, 1 in 1000), is not given by injection.

Hyperduric adrenaline is a special preparation which because of its delayed rate of absorption has a longer duration of action than ordinary adrenaline.

Other preparations include sprays, ointments and suppositories (in which it is sometimes combined with cocaine).

**Isoprenaline** (5-20 mg.) has a similar action to adrenaline and may be given either by inhalation or in the form of tablets which are allowed to dissolve under the tongue. It is frequently used in the treatment of asthma.

**Noradrenaline** (dose 2 to 8 micrograms per minute by intravenous infusion) is a hormone secreted by the adrenal medulla, also produced synthetically, which raises blood-pressure by acting as a vaso-constrictor. It is sometimes used in the treatment of shock and collapse (page 92).

'Levophed' is a preparation which may be used.

(N.B.—One ampoule contains 4 ml. of 1 in 1000 solution. 1 ml. contains the equivalent of 1 mg. of noradrenaline. One ampoule, 4 ml. is added to 1000 ml. of saline, dextrose or blood which is infused at the rate of 0·5 to 2 ml. per minute by intravenous drip.)

**Ephedrine** (*Ephedrina*), 16-60 mg. (¼ to 1 grain).

This is an alkaloid obtained from a Chinese plant, but can also be prepared by chemical means. Its action and uses are very similar to those of adrenaline. It is, however, slower and more prolonged in action and has advantages when used in some conditions. For example, it is given before a spinal anæsthetic because the rise in blood-pressure is more prolonged than that obtained by adrenaline. Unlike adrenaline, it can be given by mouth and is employed in regular doses between attacks of asthma in order to reduce their frequency.

### Ergotamine tartrate

This is an alkaloid which is extracted from ergot (a drug used for its effect on the uterus, page 208). Although it has some actions which are similar to those of adrenaline, it is not used for the same purposes but may be conveniently mentioned here. Its most important action is to constrict the blood-vessels (vaso-constriction). This may be so marked that if used in excessive doses or over a long period it may lead to gangrene of the extremities. It is sometimes used in the treatment of migraine.

It may be given (a) by injection (0·25 to 0·5 milligram), (b) by mouth (1 to 4 milligrams), when tablets should be placed under the tongue. A proprietary preparation is known as 'Femergin'.

## DRUGS ACTING LIKE PARASYMPATHETIC STIMULANTS

There are a number of drugs which have an action similar to that of the parasympathetic system. Their main actions are:

1. To stimulate the muscular movements of the bowel, i.e. to increase peristalsis. They are therefore used in conditions in which the gut is distended, e.g. post-operative distension, paralytic ileus, acute dilatation of the stomach, certain types of constipation.

2. To dilate the blood-vessels in the limbs in conditions such as Raynaud's disease. Their injection may, therefore, be associated with a fall in blood-pressure.

3. To relax the sphincter of the bladder, e.g. post-operative retention of urine.

Group I. Acetylcholine type

Acetylcholine ('Pragmoline'), 50-100 mg. ($\frac{3}{4}$ to $1\frac{1}{2}$ grains). Mecholyl, 5 to 10 milligrams approx.

**Carbachol** ('Doryl', 'Moryl'), 0·25 mg.

Group II. Anticholinesterase drugs.

**Physostigmine** (Eserine), 0·6-1·2 mg. ($\frac{1}{100}$ to $\frac{1}{50}$ grain).

This is an alkaloid which has two main uses:

(i) To relieve paralytic conditions of the bowel, e.g. post-operative distension, but drugs such as carbachol have tended to replace it.

(ii) To contract the pupil of the eye, e.g. in the treatment of glaucoma (page 211).

## Neostigmine ('Prostigmine')

This is a similar drug used especially in the treatment of myasthenia gravis. It may also be used in paralytic ileus and atony of the bladder. The dose given by mouth is about 15 milligrams, or by injection, 1 milligram.

**Pilocarpine** (*Pilocarpina*), 3-12 mg. ($\frac{1}{20}$ to $\frac{1}{5}$ grain).

This is an alkaloid obtained from a plant. It has two main actions: (i) It stimulates the secretion of sweat and saliva (pages 60, 62), (ii) it contracts the pupil of the eye.

## Drugs inhibiting action of acetylcholine (atropine group)

**Atropine** (*Atropina*), 0·25-1 mg. ($\frac{1}{240}$ to $\frac{1}{60}$ grain).

Atropine is an alkaloid obtained from the Belladonna plant (Deadly Nightshade), and the effects of belladonna preparations in the body are mainly due to the atropine which they contain. Atropine has many actions and is used for a number of therapeutic purposes.

*Action on plain muscle.* Atropine relaxes plain muscle. Thus it helps to relax the spasm of the bronchial muscle in asthma. It relaxes spasm in the muscle of the bile duct and ureter and so is of value in the treatment of biliary and renal colic.

*Action on secretions.* Atropine diminishes the secretion of the salivary glands, the sweat glands and the glands in the mucous membrane of the respiratory tract. The mouth and skin become dry and, therefore, it may be used in cases of excessive salivation and in the treatment of night sweats in pulmonary tuberculosis. (For the latter it is generally given in the form of a belladonna pill.)

Its power of diminishing the secretion of mucus from the respiratory tract is made use of in the pre-anæsthetic injection of atropine. It is also employed in the treatment of pulmonary œdema and in some cases of bronchitis.

It may be given with morphine to prevent the accumulation of bronchial secretion in the lungs, because morphine depresses the cough reflex and if an excess of mucus is present it may accumulate in the smaller bronchioles.

*Action on the stomach.* Atropine diminishes the movements of the stomach and also the amount of gastric juice secreted. It is therefore sometimes used in the treatment of gastric ulcer in the acute stages. It also tends to diminish intestinal movements and spasms and so may be given in cases of colic.

*Action on the eye* (page 210). Atropine when given by hypodermic injection or instilled into the conjunctival sac, dilates the pupils. Atropine drops are therefore employed to dilate the pupil in cases of iritis, eye injury and for purposes of examination.

*Poisoning.* Poisoning by atropine or belladonna produces the following symptoms:

1. Dryness of the mouth and throat with hoarseness of the voice.

2. Wide dilatation of the pupils.

3. Stimulation of the higher centres of the nervous system which is not apparent when therapeutic doses are used, viz. restlessness, talkativeness, delirium and often violent maniacal excitement. With large doses this stage of excitement soon passes off and is followed by depression developing into coma.

4. Skin eruptions, e.g. generalized erythema, may be present.

*Treatment:*

1. Gastric lavage.
2. Emetics, e.g. apomorphine, 6 mg., ($\frac{1}{10}$ grain) (subcutaneously).
3. Artificial respiration and oxygen.
4. Tannic acid, 20 grains in 1·2 gram in 115 ml. (4 ounces). of water, as an antidote to precipitate atropine.

### Preparation of belladonna

Tincture of belladonna (*Tinctura belladonnæ*), 2 ml. (5 to 30 minims).

For external application:

Glycerin of belladonna (*Glycerinum belladonnæ*).

Belladonna plaster (*Emplastrum belladonnæ*).

These preparations are applied externally for the relief of pain, and possibly act as counter-irritants.

## Preparations of atropine

Solution of atropine sulphate (*Liquor atropinæ sulphatis*), 0·06 ml. ($\frac{1}{2}$ to 1 minim).

Hypodermic tablets of atropine sulphate and atropine combined with morphine are available in various strengths. Most of the other preparations, e.g. ointments and drops, are used for eye conditions (page 210).

## Substances like atropine

Homatropine (page 210). Used in eye work to dilate the pupil.

Atropine methonitrate ('Eumydrin') (page 68). Used in congenital pyloric stenosis and whooping cough.

'Trasentin'. A drug having an antispasmodic action and used in renal and biliary colic.

**Hyoscine hydrobromide** (Scopolamine), 0·3-0·6 mg. ($\frac{1}{200}$ to $\frac{1}{100}$ grain).

This is one of the alkaloids obtained from hyoscyamus. Some of its actions resemble those of atropine. In addition, it depresses the central nervous system and so has an hypnotic action. It has the following uses:

1. As an hypnotic, by injection, in the treatment of mania and acute delirium, including delirium tremens, etc., although in some cases it appears to increase excitement.

2. To relieve the spasm and muscular rigidity in paralysis agitans. Like atropine, it inhibits the secretion of saliva and dryness of the mouth may be produced. This is counteracted by giving pilocarpine, 6 mg. ($\frac{1}{10}$ grain), at the same time. In this instance hyoscine is given by mouth in the form of a solution.

## Hyoscyamus

This is the dried leaf of a plant. It is mainly used for the treatment of bladder conditions. Preparations include a tincture (dose, 2-4 ml., 30-60 minims) and dry and liquid extracts.

# CHAPTER 13

# VITAMINS AND DRUGS USED IN DISORDERS OF METABOLISM

## THE VITAMINS

Vitamins or accessory food factors are substances the presence of which in the food is essential for normal health and growth.

They are found in many natural foodstuffs but, in order to maintain health, only minute quantities, compared with the bulk of other articles of diet, are required.

Our knowledge of their composition and nature has increased rapidly in recent years and it is now possible to manufacture a number of them in the laboratory. In many instances it is these synthetic products which are used in therapeutics.

It should be made clear, however, that vitamin deficiency is rare in this country and that their addition to a normal diet is rarely necessary, except perhaps in the case of infants, nursing mothers and elderly persons who may not look after themselves properly. In other words, quantities are prescribed and consumed unnecessarily.

But some special diets may be deficient in vitamins and in some diseases their absorption may not be adequate.

### Vitamin A (Axerophthol)

*Sources.* This fat-soluble vitamin is found especially in milk, butter, egg-yolk, cod-liver oil, spinach, raw carrots and other vegetables. It is probably formed in the liver from carotene, a yellow pigment found in certain vegetables.

*Effects.* Its deficiency produces:

(i) A disorder of the eyes called xerophthalmia.

(ii) Night-blindness or difficulty experienced by some people in seeing in the dark.

(iii) Roughness and dryness of the skin resulting from changes in the epithelium which may lead to diminished resistance to infection both of the skin and mucous membranes.

Vitamin A is necessary for health and growth of the young.

## Vitamin B

A number of separate substances having different actions are obtained from this group of water-soluble vitamins.

*Sources.* Most of the members of this complicated family of vitamins occur together in nature. For example they are present in the cells of both animal and vegetable tissues and are essential to the metabolic needs of the body. They are found especially in yeast, seeds (pea, bean and lentil), in eggs and in cereals such as wheat and rice. Some of the members of the group can also be prepared synthetically.

The most important are:

Vitamin $B_1$ or Aneurine, 'Thiamin.'
Vitamin $B_2$ or Riboflavine.
Vitamin $B_3$ or Nicotinic acid, Nicotinamide.
Vitamin $B_6$ or Pyridoxine.
Vitamin $B_{12}$ or Cyanocobalamin (the extrinsic anti-anæmic factor).

Other substances in this group include pantothenic acid, folic acid and biotin (vitamin H.).

## Aneurine (Vitamin $B_1$)

Severe deficiency results in beri-beri, a disease affecting the nerves (peripheral neuritis). This mainly occurs among the rice-eating populations of the East where the staple diet is polished rice.

Minor degrees of deficiency may occur either due to lack of intake or to poor absorption. The latter may take place when the normal bacterial content of the intestines is altered by the prolonged administration of antibiotics by mouth and also in chronic alcoholism.

In treatment the vitamin may be administered either by mouth or intramuscular injection (10 to 100 mg. daily).

## Riboflavine (Vitamin $B_2$)

Deficiency of this vitamin is associated with soreness of the lips and tongue and the development of fissures at the angle of the mouth. The average dose is 5 to 50 mg. daily.

| Vita-min | Names | Sources | Effects | Notes |
|---|---|---|---|---|
| **A** | *Axerophthol* | Milk butter cream egg-yolk cod-liver oil spinach tomato carrots | Raises resistance to infection Prevents night-blindness Prevents eye disease (xer-ophthalmia) | Found in vege-tables as caro-tene, probably converted into vitamin A by liver |
| **B** | *Aneurine* or *Thiamin* Anti-neuritic | Peas beans lentils wholemeal bread husks of cereals (rice, wheat, oats, barley) yeast raw carrot cabbage | Prevents beri-beri Helps in treat-ment of alco-holic neuritis | *Riboflavine* is also associated with these vitamins and is called vitamin $B_2$ *Cyanocobalamin* is vitamin $B_{12}$, the extrinsic anti-anæmic factor |
| | *Nicotinic acid* | | Prevents pel-lagra | |
| **C** | *Ascorbic acid* Anti-scor-butic | Acid fruits: orange lemon grape-fruit tomato cabbage swede | Prevents scurvy | Easily destroyed by heat and alkalis |
| **D** | *Calciferol* Anti-rachitic | Cod-liver oil eggs butter milk cream | Prevents rickets Necessary for calcium ab-sorption | Also manufac-tured in the body by the action of sun-light (ultra-violet rays) on ergosterol in the skin |
| **E** | *Tocopheryl acetate* | Wheat germ oil | ? Prevents abor-tion | — |
| **K** | *Menaphthone* | Liver spinach other vegetables | Necessary for production of prothrombin | Antidote to 'Din-devan' over-dosage $(K_1)$ |
| **P** | *Hesperidin Rutin* | Rose hips lemon juice | Effects permea-bility of capil-laries | — |

## Nicotinic acid

Pellagra, a disease causing intestinal upset, skin eruptions, nervous symptoms and mental changes is due to lack of this vitamin. This also is a tropical disease not seen in this country in its fully developed form. Nicotinic acid is sometimes used as a vaso-dilator in a number of conditions but its effect is uncertain. Doses vary from 50 to 500 mg. daily.

**Cyanocobalamin** (Vitamin $B_{12}$) is the extrinsic anti-anæmic factor used in the treatment of pernicious anæmia (page 100).

**Folic acid** is used in the treatment of sprue, cœliac disease and certain types of megalocytic anæmia. Dose 5 to 20 mg.

## Vitamin C (*Ascorbic acid*—the anti-scorbutic vitamin)

*Sources.* This is found in fresh foodstuffs, especially fruits such as oranges, lemons, black currants, rose hips, tomatoes and green vegetables, and is therefore present in salads. It is rapidly destroyed by heat and is consequently lacking in tinned foods and boiled or dried milk.

*Effects.* Deficiency results in scurvy, a disease which may affect either infants or adults. It is characterized by hæmor-rhages into the tissues, under the skin and from the gums.

Ascorbic acid may also be a factor in the formation of hæmoglobin and is sometimes given at the same time as iron in the treatment of anæmia. It can also act as a diuretic in the treatment of œdema in heart failure. It is given by mouth in doses of 50 to 100 mg. three times daily.

## Vitamin D (the anti-rachitic vitamin—*Calciferol*)

*Sources.* This is a very important vitamin and is more complicated than some of the others because it has two distinct sources:

(*a*) Its natural distribution especially in cod-liver oil (*oleum morrhuæ*), and, to some extent, in butter and eggs.

(*b*) The body is able to manufacture it for itself by the action of sunlight on a substance in the skin called ergosterol.

It is the ultra-violet rays of sunlight which have this action and, therefore, "artificial sunlight" has the same effect.

*Effects.* Lack of vitamin D causes rickets, a disease of young children characterized by deformities of the bones which are deficient in calcium. It plays an important part in the calcium metabolism of the body and its proper absorption from the intestine.

Prolonged high dosage is dangerous and may lead to the deposit of calcium in the kidneys and other organs.

The dosage varies from 1500 to 100,000 units daily.

## Vitamin E (*Tocopheryl acetate*)

This is present in the germ of wheat and its deficiency is said to result in a tendency to abortion in early pregnancy and it may possibly have some effect on the nervous system. It has no use in general medicine.

## Vitamin K (Menaphthone)

This vitamin complex which has been further subdivided into $K_1$ and $K_2$ is present in liver, spinach and other green vegetables. It is apparently necessary for the production of prothrombin (page 59) in the body and, therefore, its deficiency results in a tendency to increased bleeding. It is given in some cases of jaundice, especially before operations and in neo-natal hæmorrhage. Bile salts, which aid its absorption, are given at the same time in cases of obstructive jaundice. Synthetic preparations having the same action include menaphthone (5 to 10 milligrams by intramuscular injection) and aceto-menaphthone (10 to 60 milligrams by mouth).

**Vitamin $K_1$** (Phytonadione) acts especially as an antidote to overdosage with the anticoagulant drugs such as 'Dindevan' but not Heparin. (10 mg. are given by mouth, subcutaneously or intravenously.)

## Vitamin P

Little is known yet about this vitamin, but the functions of the capillaries appear to be influenced by it. 'Rutin' and hesperidin are similar substances.

## Vitamin Preparations

There are a number of "official" and even more proprietary vitamin preparations available. In many instances, more than one vitamin may be included in a preparation. The doses of the vitamins may be prescribed in units or by weight in milligrams.

(A) Strong capsules of vitamin A (N.F.) (*Liquor vitaminæ A fort.*), 50,000 units.

(B) Aneurine hydrochloride (*Aneurinæ hydrochloridum*), 20-50 mg., available as tablets or an injection.
  Nicotinic acid (*Acidum nicotinicum*) up to 250 milligrams.
  Riboflavine (*Lactoflavin*) up to 10 milligrams.
  'Bemax', 'Marmite', 'Benerva', 'Betaxan' and 'Becosym' are proprietary preparations containing vitamin B complex.

(C) Ascorbic acid (*Acidum ascorbicum*), up to 500 milligrams.
  Syrups of black currant and rose hips are rich sources of vitamin C, especially useful for children.

(D) Calciferol and *Liquor calciferolis*.
  Prophylactic: 0·025-0·1 mg., (1000-4000 units)
  Therapeutic: 0·125-1·25 mg. (5000-50,000 units)

(E) Tocopheryl acetate, up to 50 milligrams. 'Ephynal'.

(K) Menaphthone, 'Synkavit'.

(P) 'Hesperidin' 150 mg., 'Rutin' 20 mg.

Substances and preparations containing mixed vitamins include:

(A and D) Cod-liver oil emulsion (*Emulsio olei morrhuæ*), 8 to 30 ml.

In addition to the oil various emulsions are available which are designed to obscure its fishy taste.

Halibut liver oil capsules (*Caps. olei hippoglossi*), 1 to 3 capsules daily.

Vitamin A and D capsules (N.F.) (A = 4500, D = 450 units)

(A, B, C, and D) are contained in Vitamin Capsules (N.F.), 'Multivite'.

G

Many proprietary vitamin preparations are available but only a few have been mentioned.

Massive doses of mixed vitamin B complex with vitamin C are sometimes used in the treatment of toxic states, delirium tremens, acute alcoholism, barbiturate overdosage and acute mental conditions. Preparations for intravenous and intramuscular injection are available, e.g. 'Parentrovite'.

## DRUGS USED IN METABOLIC DISORDERS
### *Diabetes*

Diabetes is a disease due to deficiency of insulin normally secreted by the islets of Langerhans in the pancreas. It might therefore be regarded as an endocrine disorder, but its main feature is a disturbance of carbohydrate and, to some extent, fat metabolism. Normally, sugar (glucose) can only be utilized and fully oxidized by the tissues in the presence of insulin. If this is deficient, then sugar will accumulate in the blood and some of the excess will be excreted by the kidneys in the urine (glycosuria).

Further, it is only when sugar is being oxidized in the body, that an equivalent amount of fat can be fully broken down into carbon dioxide and water. If sugar is not being properly used by the tissues owing to lack of insulin, the breaking down of fat ceases at the fatty acid stage and diacetic acid and acetone (ketones) appear in the urine. The accumulation of ketones in the blood is called ketosis and ultimately leads to diabetic coma.

### Insulin

The discovery of insulin has enabled the majority of diabetics to lead a normal life and to enjoy an interesting even though restricted diet. In many cases the patient can learn to give his own injections, test his own urine, and often adjust his diet to his daily requirements. The risk of diabetic coma has been very greatly reduced, but the possibilities of insulin over-dosage must not be forgotten.

Four types of insulin are commonly employed:

1. Soluble insulin.
2. Protamine zinc insulin.
3. Globin insulin.
4. Insulin zinc suspension. (Insulin lente).

Each of these may be used alone or a dose of soluble insulin

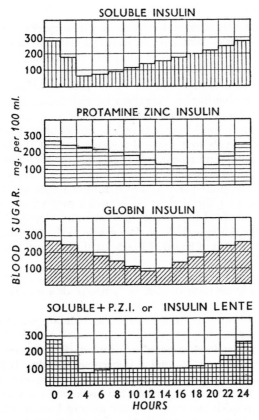

FIG. 6.—The effect of a dose of the various types of insulin in the blood sugar of a diabetic patient.

may be needed in addition to protamine zinc or globin insulin, but not to insulin zinc suspension.

**Soluble insulin** is rapidly absorbed and has its maximum effect in about four to six hours.

**Protamine zinc insulin** acts more slowly. It has little action immediately after injection, but has its greatest effect in sixteen to eighteen hours.

**Globin insulin** comes between the other two with a maximum effect at twelve hours.

**Insulin zinc suspension** (lente) is a mixture of special types of short-acting (semilente or amorphous) and long-acting (ultralente or crystalline) insulins which is administered in a single morning dose and exerts its influence over the whole 24 hours in a manner similar to the mixture of soluble and protamine zinc insulin. Insulin zinc suspension must not be mixed with other types of insulin.

The aim in every case is to reduce the number of injections to one in twenty-four hours if possible, so that the dose and type of insulin must be carefully selected for each individual.

The various types of insulin are supplied in vials containing 20, 40 or 80 units per ml., and it is most important for both the nurse and the patient to be quite sure which strength is being used. In the case of protamine zinc and globin insulin the bottle must be shaken gently so that the suspended matter is evenly diffused throughout the mixture before any is withdrawn.

A patient ordered 20 units of insulin would be given 1 ml. of ordinary strength insulin, or $\frac{1}{2}$ ml. of double strength, or $\frac{1}{4}$ ml. of quadruple strength, and so on.

The table on page 189 gives the approximate amounts to be injected when different strengths of insulin are employed.

Insulin keeps well if stored in a cool, dark place, but soluble insulin should not be used if it becomes cloudy. It may be administered with an ordinary hypodermic syringe or one specially graduated in units. This is kept in a metal case filled with spirit and may be rinsed in boiled water before use. It is wise to keep one needle for piercing the rubber cap and a separate one for injecting the insulin as the rubber is apt to

cause blunting. The top of the rubber cap having been cleansed with spirit the requisite amount of insulin is drawn into the syringe. A small amount of air injected into the insulin bottle facilitates the removal of the liquid. The skin

| Units | Single strength | | Double strength | | Quadruple strength | |
|---|---|---|---|---|---|---|
| | ml. | minims | ml. | minims | ml. | minims |
| 10 | 0·5 | 8 | 0·25 | 4 | — | — |
| 20 | 1 | 16 | 0·5 | 8 | 0·25 | 4 |
| 30 | 1·5 | 25 | 0·75 | 12 | 0·38 | 6 |
| 40 | 2 | 33 | 1 | 16 | 0·5 | 8 |
| 50 | 2·5 | 40 | 1·25 | 20 | 0·62 | 10 |
| 100 | 5 | 80 | 2·5 | 40 | 1·25 | 20 |

is cleaned with spirit or ether and the injection given sub-cutaneously. It may be made either into the arms or thighs, the latter being chosen if the patient is administering it himself. The thorax or abdominal wall may also be used, but care must be taken to select a different spot for successive injections.

Soluble insulin is given ½ hour before a meal which must contain some carbohydrate food. The other types are given before breakfast.

While the process of standardization of insulin and diet is going on, the urine must be tested for sugar and acetone before each meal. When the regular dose of insulin has been determined daily tests should be carried out on the morning specimen.

The dose of insulin generally requires to be increased if the patient is suffering from any infection (e.g. a boil, severe cold, bronchitis, etc.).

It must be clearly understood that insulin is not a cure for the disease and, once being necessary, it is probable that the patient will have to continue taking it for the rest of his life, adjustments in the dosage being required from time to time.

Because of their delayed action protamine zinc insulin, zinc suspension (lente) and globin insulin should not be used in diabetic coma.

Unless the dose is carefully adjusted, protamine zinc and globin insulin are very liable to produce hypoglycæmia.

**Other uses of insulin**

(*a*) Small doses of insulin are sometimes given in order to increase the appetite in under-nourished patients.

(*b*) Large doses are used to produce a state of shock associated with hypoglycæmia in the treatment of certain mental cases (schizophrenia).

## Oral hypoglycæmic agents

**Tolbutamide** ('Rastinon'). This substance is an oral anti-diabetic drug which lowers the blood sugar and may abolish glycosuria. Its mode of action is not clearly understood. It is most likely to be of use in an elderly diabetic in whom the disease is mild and of recent onset. In such cases the use of insulin injections may be avoided. It is unsuitable for juveniles, in diabetic coma and when there is liability to ketosis.

> Dosage: 1st day, 2-4 G.
> 2nd day, 1·5-3 G.
> 3rd day, 1-2 G.
> Subsequently, 0·5-1·5 G.

**Chlorpropamide** ('Diabinese') has a similar action and use but is given in smaller doses, viz. 250 mg. up to a maximum of 500 mg. once daily with breakfast.

Side effects such as nausea, vomiting and headache may occur and intolerance of alcohol may develop. Rarely jaundice or a skin rash is seen and indicates that the drug must be stopped at once.

### Gout

Gout is an obscure disorder of metabolism which results in the accumulation of uric acid in the blood and its deposit in the form of salts (urates) in and around joints, producing recurrent attacks of acute arthritis.

(*a*) *Used during acute attack*

## Colchicum

This is the corm of a plant. The drug relieves acute attacks

of gout but does not prevent their recurrence. It has an irritating effect on the alimentary tract, causing vomiting and purgation. It should, therefore, not be given for more than three or four days at a time.

It may be prescribed in the form of colchicum and sodium salicylate mixture (containing 1 ml. (15 minims) of tincture of colchicum in each $\frac{1}{2}$ fluid ounce). **Colchicine** tablets, each containing 1 mg. ($\frac{1}{60}$ grain) of the alkaloid colchicine are now usually employed. 1 mg. is given every two hours by mouth until the acute pain subsides.

An acute attack of gout will also respond to steroids and phenylbutazone.

*(b) Used between attacks*

Probably large doses of acetylsalicylic acid (asprin) are as effective as any other remedy. Probenecid ('Benemid'), 1-2 gram daily is also used in chronic gout.

# CHAPTER 14

# THE DUCTLESS GLANDS AND THEIR PRODUCTS

The ductless glands or endocrine organs are those glandular structures which pour their secretions (containing hormones) directly into the blood. A number of hormones have been isolated and some can be prepared in the laboratory. The functions of all the ductless glands are intimately connected with each other and also with the nervous system. The pituitary gland, in particular, exercises control over the suprarenals, thyroid, pancreas and sex glands. They play an important part in the metabolic processes of the body and in growth. Because of the balance which exists between the activities of the various glands, a disorder of one may upset the function of others.

In a broad sense, disordered function of a ductless gland may result either in an increase or a decrease in the amount of its secretion. The various ductless gland products employed in therapeutics may be used either to supply a deficiency due to under-secretion of the gland, or in order to influence the activity of other glands or organs.

The substances used may be:

   (i) The actual gland substance itself.

  (ii) Specially prepared extracts from the gland.

 (iii) Chemically prepared substances identical with or closely resembling the natural hormone.

 (iv) In certain instances, some hormones can be extracted from the urine.

## THE THYROID GLAND

The internal secretion of the thyroid is found in the colloid material secreted by the epithelium lining the vesicles of the gland. Its active principle is called thyroxine, a substance containing a high proportion of iodine (65 per cent).

Over-secretion of the thyroid gland produces thyrotoxicosis (exophthalmic goitre or Graves' disease). Among the effects of this disease is a general increase in metabolism so that the individual tends to lose weight. Under-secretion results in myxœdema in the adult, and cretinism in the infant.

Preparations of thyroid are used for the following purposes:

1. In myxœdema and cretinism, because the secretion is defective. In such cases, the patient must continue to take appropriate doses for the rest of his life.
2. In some cases of obesity, in order to increase metabolism and so produce loss of weight.

Excessive dosage produces symptoms resembling thyrotoxicosis, the most important being marked loss of weight, sweating and a rapid pulse.

## Preparations

**Thyroid** (*Thyroideum*), 30-250 mg. (½ to 4 grains) daily.

This is obtained by extracting the dried gland of animals such as oxen, sheep and pigs. It is usually supplied in tablets containing ½ grain.

Various proprietary extracts are also available, e.g. 'Elityran'. It is given by mouth and, in fact, thyroid is the only gland substance which can be given effectively in this way.

### Thyroxine sodium (0·1-0·5 mg.)

This is very powerful synthetic substance resembling the natural hormone which can be used instead of thyroid tablets. Dose: 0·05-0·5 mg. daily. A dose of 0·1 mg. is about equivalent to 60 mg. of thyroid.

### *Antithyroid substances*

In cases of thyrotoxicosis it is necessary to diminish the activity of the thyroid gland. This may be done either by surgical removal of a considerable proportion of the gland or by the administration of a drug which suppresses its activity. In any event it is usual to give some medical treatment to patients before an operation is performed.

**Iodine.** This will temporarily depress the function of the thyroid but its maximum effect is reached after two weeks of administration after which it is not maintained. It is, therefore, only suitable as a preoperative measure. Lugol's iodine (*Liquor iodi aquosus*), 0·3-1 ml. (5 to 15 minims), a watery solution of iodine with potassium, is generally employed, commencing with 2 minims and increasing to 5 or 10 minims three times a day. Potassium iodide in doses of 300 mg. daily may be used instead.

**Radioactive iodine** ($I^{131}$) may be used in the diagnosis of thyroid disease and sometimes in the treatment of thyrotoxicosis and carcinoma of the thyroid. Cases are carefully selected and an appropriate dose is required for each of the uses mentioned.

**Carbimazole.** 20-40 mg. (maintenance 5-15 mg.), 'Neomercazole'.

This is a drug which depresses the activity of the gland and can effect a medical cure of thyrotoxicosis in suitable cases. Symptoms may be controlled in one to three months but it is usually necessary to continue with a maintenance dose for six months to a year.

It is less toxic than thiouracil but may cause serious agranulocytosis and skin rashes.

**Thiouracil.** This is a sulphur-containing drug which has been used in the treatment of thyrotoxicosis in the form of methyl- or propyl-thiouracil. Although it does not have much effect on the protrusion of the eyes (exophthalmos) or the goitre, like carbimazole it restores the raised metabolism rate to normal and many patients are able to return to work after one to three months of treatment.

Toxic symptoms are sometimes produced. The most serious is diminution of the white blood cells (agranulocytosis): others include pyrexia, gland enlargement and rashes. Iodine should not be used at the same time.

**Potassium perchlorate** may also be used as an anti-thyroid drug in doses of 200 mg. four times daily. As a rule this dose may be halved after three or four weeks.

## THE PARATHYROID GLANDS

Although anatomically so closely related to the thyroid gland, the function of the parathyroids is entirely different. They secrete a hormone, the function of which is to control calcium metabolism in the body.

Deficiency of parathyroid secretion results in tetany, which is characterized by muscular spasms and increased irritability of the nervous system. The blood calcium is low. Tetany may occur, (a) after removal of the parathyroids, (b) in some cases of rickets, (c) after very large doses of alkali, (d) in sprue.

Increased activity of the parathyroids gives rise to a rare disease (osteitis fibrosa) in which there is loss of calcium from the bones.

### Preparation

**Parathyroid** (*Parathyroideum*), 3-6 mg. ($\frac{1}{20}$ to $\frac{1}{10}$ grain).

This must be given by injection. Calcium gluconate and vitamin D preparations, e.g. Calciferol, 100,000 units daily, are sometimes given at the same time. A substance called dihydrotachysterol ('A.T. 10') chemically related to vitamin D and resembling parathyroid hormone in action, may be given by mouth in doses of 1-3 mg. (3 to 10 ml.) for tetany.

## THE SUPRARENAL OR ADRENAL GLANDS

The two suprarenal glands consist of an outer cortex and central medulla each of which produce hormones differing in chemical character and function. The glands are plentifully supplied with blood and also with sympathetic nerve fibres from the cœliac (solar) plexus.

### The functions of the cortex

The suprarenal cortex is essential to life and secretes a number of hormones, each having different functions. Some of these have been extracted from the gland and some can be made in the laboratory.

Chemically they belong to a class of fatty or wax-like substances called steroids or corticoids. The most important ones fall into three main groups:

1. The ***Mineral Corticoids*** of which deoxycortone (DOCA) and aldosterone are examples. These act on the tubules of the kidney in such a way that:

(a) sodium and chloride are retained in the body.

(b) excess of potassium is excreted.

They therefore help to maintain the water and electrolyte balance of the body. Any excess or overdosage will lead to water retention (œdema) and hypertension.

2. The *Gluco-corticoids* or *Corticosteroids*. This group includes cortisone and its derivatives. (For brevity the term "steroid" may be employed.) These hormones have a number of actions, one of the main ones being to influence carbohydrate and glucose metabolism.

(a) They assist in the conversion of carbohydrate into glycogen.

(b) They increase the blood sugar.

(c) They help in the utilization of fat.

(d) They decrease the number of lymphocytes and eosinophils in the blood.

(e) They reduce the rate at which certain connective tissue cells multiply and so tend to suppress the natural reaction to inflammation and to delay healing.

(f) They increase the secretion of hydrochloride acid in the stomach, thus tending to cause peptic ulcers or to delay their healing.

(g) In large doses cortisone produces symptoms similar to Cushing's syndrome, viz. a swollen, round 'moon face', excess of hair and a tendency to acne.

(h) Electrolyte and water metabolism disturbances.

3. *Sex or Gonad-like Hormones* similar to those produced by the ovary and testis (œstrogens and androgens). These influence growth and sex development.

The output of hormones from the cortex of the suprarenal is controlled by another hormone secreted by the pituitary gland known as the adreno-cortico-trophic hormone (ACTH) or corticotrophin. Unlike the medulla of the suprarenal the secretions of the cortex are not regulated by nervous impulses.

Cortisone, hydrocortisone and two similar synthetic substances (prednisone and prednisolone) are all used in clinical medicine. When these are administered in large or excessive doses among the complications observed is a disturbance of salt and water balance, which is, as mentioned above, a function of the mineral corticoids and not of the gluco-corticoids.

The explanation of this apparent paradox is that large doses of cortisone, in addition to the normal actions mentioned, also depress the secretion of corticotrophin (ACTH) from the pituitary.

Deficiency of corticotrophin (ACTH) will, therefore, result in alteration of the secretion of the mineral corticoids and so upset the salt and water balance.

It must also be remembered that although the individual hormones mentioned each have separate effects on metabolism, in health, normal suprarenal cortical secretion represents the sum of all these individual actions.

In disease, if the suprarenal cortex is destroyed or if the secretion of corticotrophin (ACTH) fails there will be no suprarenal cortical hormones produced.

### Mineral corticoids

1. **Deoxycortone** (DOCA), 2-5 mg. This mineral corticoid which causes water and sodium retention is mainly used in conjunction with cortisone in the treatment of Addison's disease. Overdosage produces œdema and hypertension.

(a) It may be given by intramuscular injection in doses of 2-5 mg. daily.

(b) Pellets (100-400 mg.) may be implanted under the skin whence it is slowly absorbed over a period of about six months.

### Gluco-corticoids (Corticosteroids)

2. **Cortisone** 50-200 mg. Since cortisone was originally discovered a number of other substances having a similar general action have been made by varying slightly its chemical composition. By means of these variations it has been possible to minimize some of the side effects so that prednisone and prednisolone cause less salt and water retention and can be given in one fifth of the dose of cortisone.

Hydrocortisone is the form in which the hormone is actually secreted in the body by the adrenal glands and its action is identical with that of cortisone.

There are a large number of proprietary preparations of

these substances each having different names and too numerous to mention here.

The cortisone group of drugs may be used as tablets, injections, ointments and eye drops.

(*a*)  Cortisone, prednisone and prednisolone are used mainly for internal administration.

(*b*)  Hydrocortisone, although it can be given internally and, in grave emergency, by intravenous injection, is used mainly for local application and local injection into and around joints.

**Cortisone** (50-200 mg.), **prednisone and prednisolone** (5-50 mg. daily)

These substances may be used either as direct replacement therapy, i.e. to replace the natural hormone when the secretion of the adrenal gland is defective as in Addison's disease or after removal of both glands (which may be performed for certain cases of carcinoma, e.g. of the breast) or empirically, where increase of the cortical steroid hormones have been shown by experiment to be beneficial.

Among the many conditions in which they may be used are:

1.  *Rheumatic and collagen diseases.*

    Rheumatic fever              polyarteritis nodosa
    rheumatoid arthritis         lupus erythematosus
    acute gout

2.  *Allergic disorders.*

    severe asthma                drug sensitivity
    status asthmaticus           serum sickness

3.  *Skin diseases.*

    pemphigus vulgaris           dermatitis
    erythema multiforme

4.  *Endocrine disorders.*

    Addison's disease            pituitary disorders
    adrenalectomy

5.  *Blood diseases.*

    hæmolytic anæmia             purpura

6.  *Other disorders.*

    ulcerative colitis           temporal arteritis
    burns                        sarcoidosis
    nephrotic syndrome           delirium tremens

There are a number of other uncommon conditions in which the use of cortisone may be considered desirable. It must be understood, however, that it is only used in selected cases and is not necessarily employed in every case of the diseases listed.

*Contraindications.* Being a very powerful drug cortisone must be used with great caution and under careful supervision. It is usually contraindicated in the presence of peptic ulcer, hypertension and cardiac insufficiency, and in most cases of active or old tuberculosis although there are special indications for its use in some cases of tuberculosis.

In view of the fact that the administration of cortisone tends to inhibit the natural secretion from the adrenal gland while it is being given the drug should be withdrawn gradually over a period of one to two weeks when therapy has been completed otherwise serious withdrawal symptoms may occur.

When cortisone is given in large doses the following observations are desirable:

(*a*)  Daily weight, urinary output and blood pressure records.

(*b*)  Observation for œdema, "moon face" and thrombophlebitis of legs.

(*c*)  Diet: high protein, restricted fat and carbohydrate.

(*d*)  Drugs: potassium chloride to prevent potassium depletion;
aluminium hydroxide to prevent peptic ulcer;
antibiotics in the presence of infection;
sedatives to minimize mental disturbances.

These precautions are unnecessary when prednisone and prednisolone are used unless large doses are employed.

**Hydrocortisone.** This may be injected with strict aseptic precautions into or around joints. Doses of 0·25-1 ml. (25 mg. per ml.) are used according to the size of the joint or area to be infiltrated.

Among the conditions for which it may be employed are:

| | |
|---|---|
| rheumatoid arthritis | traumatic arthritis |
| osteoarthritis | "tennis elbow" |
| periarthritis | acute gout |
| bursitis | keloid scars |

Retention enemas may be given in ulcerative colitis, e.g. 50-100 mg. in 5 oz. of 1 per cent methyl cellulose emulsion or normal saline once or twice daily.

### Hydrocortisone lotion and skin ointment

Lotions are generally used for wet surfaces and extensive lesions, ointments for dry localized lesions and those near the eyes. At first applications may be made up to four times daily and later reduced to daily or alternate days. Among the indications are:

| | |
|---|---|
| allergic skin disorders | pruritus |
| eczema of various types | contact dermatitis |

### Hydrocortisone eye drops (1%) and eye ointment (2·5%)

| | |
|---|---|
| blepharitis | interstitial keratitis |
| conjunctivitis | iritis |

Their use is contraindicated in acute corneal ulcer.

## Functions of adrenal medulla

The medulla secretes adrenaline, the properties of which have already been mentioned (page 173); they include:

(i) It is a general stimulant of the sympathetic system.

(ii) It is a vaso-constrictor.

(iii) It raises blood-pressure.

(iv) It causes the liver to liberate glycogen.

The medulla also secretes noradrenaline, a natural hormone closely related to adrenaline which can also be prepared synthetically. It also raises blood pressure by vasoconstriction but has little effects on the bronchial muscle.

In Addison's disease, which is usually due to tuberculosis of the suprarenal glands, both the cortex and medulla are involved. It is characterized by low blood-pressure, digestive disturbances, general weakness and a brown pigmentation of the skin. There is loss of sodium from the blood, and loss of fluid from the tissues (dehydration) may be marked, i.e. the electrolyte and fluid balance is disturbed.

## THE PITUITARY GLAND

This consists of two parts which have different modes of development and entirely different functions.

1. *Anterior lobe.* This secretes a number of hormones having the following functions:

(*a*) The growth hormone (somatotrophin).

(*b*) The thyrotrophic hormone (TTH). This appears to stimulate the growth and activity of the thyroid gland and to increase the basal metabolic rate.

(*c*) The adreno-cortico-trophic hormone (ACTH). This hormone is a protein substance which stimulates the cortex of the suprarenal gland to secrete its own hormones, e.g.:

    (i) Mineral steroids (corticoids) e.g. deoxycortone (DOCA) and aldosterone.

    (ii) Gluco-steroids e.g. cortisone, etc. (see page 196).

(*d*) The gonado-trophic hormones (GTH). These are essential for the normal development of the sex organs and stimulate the production of the various sex gland hormones. They are:

    (i) The follicle stimulating hormone (FSH). In the female this stimulates the ovarian follicles to produce œstrogen. In the male it stimulates the production of spermatozoa.

    (ii) The luteinizing hormone (LH). In the female this stimulates the corpus luteum of the ovary to produce progesterone. In the male, the testes to produce testosterone.

(*e*) The lactogenic hormone (prolactin) which helps to control the secretion of milk from the breast.

(*f*) There are other hormones which affect sugar and fat metabolism, disturbances of which may lead to glycosuria and ketosis, and hormones which affect the functions of the parathyroid glands and the pancreas.

### Adreno-cortico-trophic hormone (ACTH), corticotrophin

ACTH is a hormone obtained from the anterior lobe of the pituitary gland used in therapeutics. Its action is to stimulate the cortex of the suprarenal gland to produce various hormones, the most important of which is cortisone.

The effect of cortisone can, therefore, be produced either by its own direct administration or by giving ACTH which stimulates its production in the body.

They may be used in diseases affecting the respective glands, i.e. ACTH is given in hypopituitarism and cortisone in Addison's disease.

They also have effects in many other conditions, although the use of cortisone or one of its preparations is generally preferred to ACTH.

ACTH is given by intramuscular injection in doses of 10 to 25 units at six hourly intervals. Gelatin preparations which delay absorption are also available so that only a daily injection is necessary.

### Anterior lobe preparations

Apart from ACTH it has not been found possible to prepare individual hormones for therapeutic use from the anterior lobe. Various proprietary extracts from the anterior lobe are sometimes used in certain disorders of growth.

Substances having an action on the gonads or sex glands similar to that produced by the anterior pituitary hormones can be obtained from the placenta and urine of pregnant women and mares. These are called *gonadotrophic hormones* and are sometimes used in the treatment of menorrhagia, dysmenorrhœa and sterility in the female. In the male they may be used for undescended testicle and some cases of impotence. In all cases their effects are variable and uncertain.

1. Chorionic Gonadotrophin (from urine of pregnant women).

Dose: 500-1000 units, twice weekly, intramuscularly. Proprietary preparations include 'Pregnyl', 'Gonan'. The action resembles LH.

2. Serum Gonadotrophin (from serum of pregnant mares). Dose: 200-1000 units, twice weekly, intramuscularly. The action resembles a mixture of LH and FSH.

### Posterior lobe preparations

Extracts of the posterior lobe which contain two active substances:

1. **Oxytocin** ('Pitocin'). This is only used in obstetrics, to

cause contraction of the uterus during and just after labour without increasing the blood-pressure.

(i) In the second stage of labour, when the os is fully dilated, to overcome uterine inertia.

(ii) In the treatment of post-partum hæmorrhage.

(iii) To aid the expulsion of the placenta or retained products from the uterus after delivery.

(iv) To stimulate uterine contraction during the operation of Cæsarean section, immediately after the infant and the placenta have been removed. In this instance it is sometimes injected directly into the uterine muscle.

Dose: Injection of oxytocin (B.P.) 2-5 units.

2. **Vasopressin** ('Pitressin') which has the following actions:

(*a*) To raise blood pressure by acting on the plain muscles of the arteries producing vaso-constriction.

(*b*) To cause contraction of plain muscle, especially of the intestines and bladder.

(*c*) An anti-diuretic action causing water retention in the body. Use is made of this property in the treatment of diabetes insipidus, in which it may be administered by injection or in the form of snuff.

Dose: Injection of vasopressin (B.P.) 2-5 units.

*'Pituitrin'* is a proprietary preparation containing both substances and therefore has the following actions:

(*a*) Those due to oxytocin ('Pitocin')—see above.

(*b*) Those due to vasopressin ('Pitressin') which stimulates plain muscle:

(i) It increases peristalsis in the intestines and is used in cases of paralytic ileus and post-operative distension.

(ii) To cause vaso-constriction by acting on the plain muscle in the arteries and so to raise blood-pressure. Hence its value in shock and collapse.

(iii) On account of other actions it is sometimes used in diabetes insipidus, hæmoptysis, herpes zoster.

## THE SEX GLANDS

The hormones used in therapy may be divided into two main groups:

1. Female sex hormones derived from the ovary.

2. Male sex hormones derived from the testis.

Some synthetic preparations are also available.

### 1. The internal secretions of the ovary

Two main types of preparation are used:

(a) Œstrogens

(b) Progesterone

### (a) Œstrogens

These are substances which produce the effects of the hormone of the ovarian follicle including:

(i) Development of the female secondary sexual characteristics, i.e. growth of pubic and axillary hair, the breasts and external genitalia.

(ii) Rhythmic contraction of the Fallopian tube and its fimbriæ which collect the ovum at the time of ovulation.

(iii) Growth of the uterine muscle and endometrium.

(iv) Secretion from the glands of the cervix.

(v) The smoothness of the female skin in comparison with the greasy skin of the male.

The main uses are:

(i) To diminish unpleasant symptoms occurring at the menopause.

(ii) To suppress lactation on weaning or after a stillbirth.

(iii) In certain cases of excessive uterine bleeding (metropathia hæmorrhagica).

(iv) In some cases of amenorrhœa.

(v) In senile vaginitis and kraurosis vulvæ.

(vi) In some cases of carcinoma of the prostate in males and of the breast in females.

(vii) In some cases of acne both in the male and female.

Toxic effects include:

(i) Nausea and vomiting.

(ii) Excessive uterine bleeding especially after the drug is withdrawn.

There are two main types of œstrogen:

(i) Natural: obtained from human sources or from the urine of pregnant mares: e.g. œstrone, œstradiol, premarin.

(ii) Synthetic: e.g. stilbœstrol, dienœstrol, ethinylœstradiol, methallenœstril.

Generally speaking the former are expensive and the latter relatively cheap (especially stilbœstrol).

The doses vary according to the preparation and the purpose for which it is given. Oral administration is usually effective but preparations for intramuscular injection are available. Many proprietary preparations are on the market. Menopax cream, used locally for pruritus vulvæ, contains stilbœstrol, amethocaine and benzocaine.

'Conovid' is a proprietary preparation which may be used for fertility control.

## (b) Progesterone

This is a hormone formed mainly by the cells of the corpus luteum which develop in the ovarian follicle after the ovum has been extruded. Its main action is to sensitize the endometrium and prepare it for the reception of the fertilized ovum. It also relaxes plain muscle, which may contribute to the occurrence of varicose veins, constipation and dilatation of the ureters during pregnancy.

Its main use is when combined with œstrogen in the treatment of menstrual disorders and in the treatment of excessive uterine bleeding. Its effects in the treatment of abortion and sterility are uncertain. Preparations are given by intramuscular injection in the form of an oily solution.

Ethisterone, a synthetic preparation, may be given by mouth but about five times the dose of progesterone is required.

## 2. *The male sex hormones* (Androgens)

**Testosterone**

This is an active substance which is obtained from the testes and which can also be prepared chemically.

Various compounds of testosterone may be given by intramuscular injection or by implantation under the skin. Methyltestosterone is given by mouth.

Other drugs of the androgen type include norethandrolone ('Nilevar') and nandrolone ('Durabolin').

Main uses:

1. Male hypogonadism and after castration.
2. In a number of gynæcological conditions including excessive uterine bleeding, endometriosis and premenstrual tension.

Testosterone may produce excessive growth of facial hair in the female and salt and water retention leading to œdema.

# CHAPTER 15

## MISCELLANEOUS DRUGS

### DRUGS ACTING ON THE UTERUS

The uterus is an organ composed of plain muscle-fibres and lined by a special type of mucous membrane, the endometrium. Its functions are (i) to receive the fertilized ovum and to retain the developing fœtus throughout pregnancy, (ii) to expel the fœtus and placenta at the termination of pregnancy.

After puberty the endometrium undergoes a series of periodic changes by which it is prepared to receive a fertilized ovum at regular intervals of about a month. Menstruation is the process by which the specially prepared endometrium is shed when no fertilized ovum has been received.

When the end of pregnancy is reached, the greatly hypertrophied muscle of the body of the uterus commences to contract in a succession of recurring spasms which gradually increase in frequency. At the same time the muscle of the cervix dilates, and when fully dilated the head of the fœtus can descend to the perineum, whence the child is finally delivered. Some minutes later this is followed by the placenta and the membranes which surround the fœtus during its development in the uterus.

Apart from the female sex hormones which may influence ovarian and uterine function, comparatively few drugs have any important action on the non-pregnant uterus.

### *Drugs which increase uterine contraction*

The drugs which increase uterine contraction once labour is due or has commenced are called ECBOLICS.

There are no drugs which act on the uterus in the early stages of pregnancy which would cause it to expel its contents without producing poisonous symptoms dangerous to the life of the mother. In other words, there are no true abortifacients which have any therapeutic use. If, for medical reasons, it is necessary to terminate pregnancy in the early stages, operative procedures must be carried out.

### Ergot (*Ergota*)

This is a fungus which grows on rye and sometimes on other kinds of grain. Its action is due to the various alkaloids which it contains. It causes contraction of the muscle of the pregnant uterus during and after labour, and is, therefore, especially valuable:

(i) In the treatment of post-partum hæmorrhage, when the contraction of the uterine muscle closes the bleeding vessels.

(ii) In aiding the expulsion of the placenta and any retained products of conception.

(iii) To keep the uterine muscle firmly contracted during the first few days of the puerperium.

The following preparations may be employed:

Ergometrine maleate

Ergot capsules and tablets, 150-500 mg. ($2\frac{1}{2}$-$7\frac{1}{2}$ grains).

*Ergometrine Maleate.* This is an alkaloid which is given in the following doses:

By mouth (tablets): 0·5-1 mg. ($\frac{1}{120}$-$\frac{1}{60}$ grain).

By intramuscular injection: 0·25-1 mg. ($\frac{1}{240}$-$\frac{1}{60}$ grain).

By intravenous injection: 0·125-0·5 mg. ($\frac{1}{480}$-$\frac{1}{120}$ grain).

*Ergotoxine*, another alkaloid, 0·5-1 mg. ($\frac{1}{100}$ to $\frac{1}{50}$ grain).

### Pituitary (*Posterior lobe*)

It has already been noted (page 200) that the extract of the posterior lobe of the pituitary contains oxytocin ('Pitocin') which causes the plain muscle of the pregnant uterus to contract without producing a rise in blood-pressure. Subcutaneous or intramuscular dose, 2 to 5 units.

Pituitary (posterior lobe) Injection, B.P.C., 0·2-0·5 ml.

### Quinine (*Quinina*)

Quinine is a drug having a number of actions (page 218). Among them is the ability to cause labour to commence during the last weeks of pregnancy.

It is therefore used in the "medical induction" of premature labour in the following way:

7 a.m. Castor oil, 1 to 2 ounces.

8 a.m. Hot bath.

9 a.m. Enema, after which a tight abdominal binder is applied.

10 a.m. to 4 p.m. Two-hourly doses of quinine bi-hydrochloride, 5 grains.

9 p.m. If pains have not commenced, 2 units of 'Pituitrin' which may be repeated every half hour for 8 doses.

### Uterine sedatives

These are substances which diminish the force and frequency of the muscular contractions of the pregnant uterus, e.g.

Morphine          Chloral hydrate

### Diagnosis of uterine conditions

Lipiodol (iodized oil) may be injected into the uterine cavity. Normally, it fills this cavity and also the Fallopian tubes. An X-ray after the injection shows the outline of the uterus, its size and shape and also the patency of the tubes. This procedure may be of importance in the diagnosis of sterility and is called a "uterogram".

### Preparations acting on the Vagina

1. Trichomonas infection: acetarsol pessaries.
2. Monilia infections: Crystal Violet pessaries. Nystatin.
3. Antiseptic application: (*a*) Chloroxylenol irrigation, one tablespoonful of solution mixed with one pint of warm water, (*b*) Proflavine pessaries.
4. Astringent lotions: Zinc Sulphate irrigation. 90 grains in one pint of warm water (6 gram in 500 ml.).
5. To alter acidity of Vagina: Lactic Acid pessary, Lactic Acid irrigation. One teaspoonful in one pint warm water.
6. For senile vaginitis: Stilbœstrol pessary.

## DRUGS ACTING ON THE EYE

Therapeutic substances may be applied to the eyes in the following types of preparation:

Eye lotions (*Collyria*). ⎫
Eye drops (*Guttæ pro oculis*). ⎪  For details see National
Eye ointments (*Oculenta*). ⎬        Formulary.
Gelatin discs (*Lamellæ*). ⎭

### I. Drugs which dilate the pupil
### (Mydriatics)

The most important are atropine and homatropine.

### Atropine

Atropine dilates the pupil and paralyses the power of accommodation when given internally and when applied locally to the eye (page 178). Locally, it takes several hours to produce its full effect, which lasts for several days. It has the disadvantage of increasing the tension within the eye and is, therefore, contra-indicated in cases of glaucoma. It is used for the following purposes:

(i) In the treatment of iritis. By paralysing its power of movement the iris is rested.
(ii) In cases of corneal ulcer.
(iii) In injury to the eyeball.
(iv) For purposes of examination of the retina.

It may be applied in the form of drops, gelatin discs or an ointment.

Atropine sulphate drops (*Guttæ atropinæ sulphatis*), 1 per cent.
Atropine discs (*Lamellæ atropinæ*), 0·065 mg. ($\frac{1}{5000}$ grain).
Atropine eye ointment (*Oculentum atropinæ*), 0·25 per cent.

These preparations are sometimes combined with cocaine for use in painful conditions.

### Homatropine

This has a similar but much more rapid, though less prolonged, action than atropine. The pupils are dilated in 5 to 15 minutes and the effect passes off in a few hours.

Homatropine is especially useful for rapid dilatation of the pupils prior to examination of the optic discs.

Drops (2%) or gelatine discs may be employed. Ointments are also available, and cocaine may be added for the treatment of painful conditions.

NORMAL

MORPHINE
(pin point)

MYOTIC
e.g. Physostigmine
(Eserine)

MYDRIATIC
e.g. Atropine
Cocaine
Adrenaline

FIG. 7—Diagram illustrating the action of drugs on the pupil.

It must be remembered that patients may not be able to see properly until the effects of atropine and homatropine have worn off. Reading will be impossible and they may find it very difficult to get about out of doors in bright light.

## II. Drugs which contract the pupil
## (Myotics)

**Physostigmine** (Eserine)

This is the most important myotic drug. It is used especially in the treatment of glaucoma and may be employed to counteract the effect of atropine and homatropine when eye examinations have been completed. In glaucoma, contraction of the iris helps to open up the lymph channels in the ciliary body, thereby facilitating the drainage of fluid from the interior of the eye and lowering intra-ocular tension. (See also page 176.)

Drops, gelatine discs and ointment may be used:

Physostigmine or eserine drops (*Guttæ physostigminæ*), 0·5 per
**cent.**

Physostigmine or eserine discs (*Lamellæ physostigminæ*), ·065 mg. ($\frac{1}{1000}$ grain).

Physostigmine or eserine eye ointment (*Oculentum physostigminæ*) (0·125 per cent).

## Local anæsthetics

**Cocaine** drops, 2 per cent are generally employed. (*a*) For operations on the eye, (*b*) to render the conjunctiva anæsthetized in order that a foreign body may be removed and (*c*) in the treatment of painful conditions.

## Antiseptic eye drops and ointments

These are used in the treatment of various types of conjunctivitis and corneal ulceration. Silver preparations have been employed in the prophylaxis and treatment of ophthalmia neonatorum.

Silver protein (*Guttæ argentoproteini mitis*, Argyrol drops).
Zinc sulphate, 0·25 per cent (*Guttæ zinci sulphatis*).
Streptomycin.
Sulphacetamide, 'Albucid', 10 per cent (*Guttæ sulphacetamidi*).
Penicillin (*Guttæ penicillini*).⎫          eye drops
Chloramphenicol ('Chloromycetin').⎬          and
Hydrocortisone.⎭          ointments

**Castor oil** is sometimes instilled into the conjunctiva in cases of corneal abrasion. It is also used after anæsthesia with chloroform or ether, to prevent subsequent inflammation due to the irritation of their vapour.

**Fluorescein** (*Guttæ fluoresceini*, 2 per cent), placed in the conjunctival sac, stains corneal abrasions and ulcers and makes them clearly visible.

## DRUGS USED IN THE TREATMENT OF SYPHILIS

Syphilis is a disease caused by the *Spirochæta pallida* (*Treponema pallidum*). Its clinical manifestations occur in three stages:

I. The primary sore or chancre.

II. The secondary stage, commencing about 6 weeks after infection and lasting up to 2 years, during which skin rashes and various other symptoms may arise.

III. The tertiary stage in which gummata are found. The cardio-vascular system, bones or nervous system may be affected.

Congenital syphilis may also occur.

The routine treatment of syphilis is to give a full course of Penicillin (e.g. 1 million units daily for ten days) or one of the other antibiotics (page 235). Further treatment is controlled by the results of the Wasserman reaction. In some cases of tertiary syphilis a course of bismuth injections may be given before penicillin is commenced. Potassium iodide is also sometimes given by mouth. Arsenic and mercury preparations are now rarely employed.

### Organic arsenic compounds

There are a number of organic arsenic compounds of complicated chemical composition which were formerly used in the treatment of syphilis. The first to be used was Arsphenamine or Salvarsan (606), which was discovered by Ehrlich in the early years of this century. This drug was given by intravenous drip methods, but the preparation of the solution and its administration was complicated and it was replaced by other drugs which were easier to handle.

**Neoarsphenamine,** 0·15 to 0·9 gram. This is also known as Novarsenobenzol, N.A.B., etc. It is a yellow powder, readily soluble in water. Leakage of the drug under the skin is liable to cause severe inflammation and, for this reason it is only given intravenously.

A typical course of 8 to 10 injections would consist of 0·45 gram, followed by doses of 0·6 gram and later, 0·75 gram at weekly intervals until a total of 5 grams had been given.

**Sulpharsphenamine,** 0·1 to 0·6 gram. This is also known as 'Sulfarsenol', 'Sulphostab', etc. It has the advantage that it can be given by intramuscular injection without risk of producing local inflammation.

**Tryparsamide,** 1 to 2 grams. This is an arsenical preparation which can be given either by intramuscular or intravenous injection. It was originally introduced for the treatment of sleeping sickness (a tropical disease due to *Trypanosoma gambiense*, which must not be confused with encephalitis lethargica, sometimes called "sleepy sickness"). There is a risk of producing damage to the optic nerve leading to blindness (optic atrophy).

In addition to their use in syphilis, the organic arsenic compounds have been employed in the treatment of (*a*) Vincent's angina (a single dose of 0·3 gram of neoarsphenamine being usually sufficient to cure the disease), and (*b*) anthrax.

Sulpharsphenamine is sometimes used in disseminated sclerosis.

## Toxic symptoms

Certain toxic symptoms may result from the therapeutic use of arsenical compounds, including:

- (i) Collapse immediately after injection, which is treated by the injection of 1 ml. adrenaline, 1 in 1000.
- (ii) Rigors and headache.
- (iii) Severe generalized dermatitis, treated by injection of dimercaprol (B.A.L.).
- (iv) Jaundice, treated by intravenous glucose and calcium gluconate.

**'Devegan' vaginal tablets** and **Acetarsol vaginal compound** (S.V.C.) contain organic arsenic compounds and they are used in cases of vaginal discharge (leucorrhœa), especially that due to infection with *Trichomonas vaginalis*.

## Inorganic arsenic

A few inorganic arsenic compounds have been used in general medicine such as Arsenical solution (*Liquor arsenicalis*, Fowler's solution) 0·5 ml. (2 to 8 minims). It is given internally as a general tonic, usually in mixture form with iron (*Mistura ferri arsenicalis*), but its value is doubtful, and in recent years it has tended to fall into disuse. Inorganic arsenic has no effect in syphilis.

## Poisoning by inorganic arsenic

This may be suicidal or homicidal. Arsenic is present in many weed-killers, in which form it is most easily obtained. The symptoms depend on the dosage taken. A large dose produces epigastric pain, vomiting, diarrhœa, excessive thirst, muscular cramps and collapse which may soon terminate fatally. Smaller doses given over a longer period result in loss of appetite, intermittent attacks of diarrhœa, thirst, colicky abdominal pains, pigmentation of the skin and symptoms of peripheral neuritis such as wrist-drop, numbness and loss of tendon reflexes. Arsenic remains in the body for some time and can be recovered from the hair, nails, liver and other organs.

## Mercury (*Hydrargyrum*)

Mercury or quicksilver (having the chemical symbol of Hg) is an element which has the form of a bright liquid metal.

It is used in thermometers, and also in the sphygmomano-meter and other types of pressure gauge. The metal itself is an ingredient of a number of preparations used in medicine. Mercury salts are also employed. Mersalyl and 'Neptal', are organic compounds of mercury. Mercury preparations have a number of actions on the body.

### (1) External application

(a) *Antiseptic.* Mercuric chloride (*Hydrargyri perchloridum*, corrosive sublimate) and mercury biniodide are used as anti-septics (page 40). Mercurochrome and thiomersal ('Merthio-late') are organic mercurial compounds used for external application in the form of solutions, paints, ointments, etc.

(b) *Antiseptic and antiparasitic ointments.* There are a number of ointments containing mercury used, for example, in the treatment of impetigo and pediculosis pubis, e.g. ammoniated mercury ointment.

Oxide of mercury eye ointment, Golden eye ointment (*oculentum hydrargyri oxidi flavum*) is sometimes used for con-junctivitis and blepharitis.

(c) *Counter-irritants.* The stronger mercury ointments, e.g. Scott's dressing (*Unguentum hydrargyri compositum*), may be used in the treatment of synovitis or injured joints.

Some people show special skin sensitivity to mercury, and its application in any form may be followed by a rash.

### (2) Internal administration

(a) *On the alimentary tract.* With large doses the flow of saliva is increased and, if taken over a long period, the mouth and gums become inflamed (stomatitis). Irritation of the intestine is also caused and it will be recalled that calomel has been used as a purgative (page 75).

(b) *On the kidneys.* Certain mercury preparations, especially mersalyl, are diuretics and increase the flow of urine.

### Mercurial poisoning

The acute symptoms include stomatitis, with a metallic taste in the mouth, gastro-enteritis (diarrhœa and vomiting), and nephritis (blood and albumin in the urine), followed by collapse in serious cases. In chronic cases, in addition to any of the above, peripheral neuritis may develop.

## Bismuth (*Bismuthum*)

Bismuth is employed therapeutically both in its metallic state and in the form of various salts.

**Metallic bismuth.** Prepared in the form of finely divided particles, may be given by the intramuscular injection of a suspension in glucose solution (*Injectio bismuthi*, 1 ml., 8 to 15 minims), in the treatment of syphilis.

Bismuth salts by mouth have no effect in the treatment of syphilis but are used for various other purposes.

### External application

**Bismuth subgallate** ('Dermatol'). This is sometimes used as a dusting powder and ointment in skin conditions.

Bismuth and iodoform paste (BIPP), see page 46.

### Internal administration

**Bismuth carbonate** (*Bismuthi carbonas*, bismuth oxy-carbonate), 2 gram (10 to 30 grains), is sometimes used as a weak antacid and gastric sedative in cases of gastritis and gastric ulcer. It is also used in diarrhœa.

## DRUGS USED IN THE TREATMENT OF MALARIA

Malaria is essentially a disease acquired in the tropics and caused by the malarial parasite which is introduced into the body by the bite of an infected Anopheles mosquito. Each parasite gains entrance to a red blood corpuscle where it multiplies and, when a new generation is fully formed, the young parasites are discharged from the red cells into the blood-stream in which they circulate freely until each again enters a red corpuscle. This process is repeated indefinitely. The infected red corpuscles degenerate and are destroyed by the spleen, which becomes enlarged.

The characteristic feature of the disease is the occurrence of rigors at regular intervals of 48 to 72 hours, according to the species of parasite present. The occurrence of rigors coincides with a fresh generation of young parasites being liberated from the red corpuscles.

## Anti-malarial drugs

For many years quinine was the only drug used in the prevention and treatment of malaria. It has now been largely replaced by various synthetic products, e.g.

Proguanil ('Paludrine')
Chloroquine
Pamaquin ('Plasmoquine')
Mepacrine ('Atebrin')

Anti-malarial drugs may be given:

(a) *Prophylactically.* It is a usual practice for persons living in malaria-infested districts to take regular doses of an anti-malarial drug in order to prevent the disease if they happen to be bitten by an infected mosquito.

The most effective are:

Pamaquin in daily doses of 100 mg.

Chloroquine preparations in weekly doses of 300 mg.

(b) *Treatment of an attack*

Chloroquine preparations, 600 mg., followed by 300 mg. daily for two days.

Mepacrine in doses of 200 to 500 mg. daily.

In cerebral malaria and other serious types chloroquine may be given by intramuscular injection or by intravenous drip. Quinine can also be given intravenously but intramuscular injection is likely to cause abscess formation.

New anti-malarial substances are being manufactured and tested.

**Pamaquin** ('Plasmoquine'), 25-50 mg. ($\frac{2}{5}$ to $\frac{4}{5}$ grain).

This is a synthetic drug which is useful in prophylaxis and also in the after-treatment of the disease to prevent relapses. It is rarely employed in the acute stages and its prolonged administration is sometimes accompanied by cyanosis and collapse.

**Mepacrine** ('Atebrin'), 50-100 mg. ($\frac{3}{4}$ to $1\frac{1}{2}$ grains).

Another synthetic drug which may produce a harmless

H

yellow coloration of the skin. o·1 gram, three times a day for 7 days, may be given in the treatment of an acute attack. It is generally given orally, but in serious cases and in cerebral malaria it is suitable for intramuscular injection.

This drug is also given by mouth in the treatment of tape worms.

N.B. The real prophylaxis of malaria is to destroy the breeding grounds of the mosquito by draining stagnant water or preventing the hatching of the larva into the adult mosquito by covering such pools with paraffin. A bed net to prevent bites at night is also essential.

## Quinine (*Quinina*)

Quinine is an alkaloid obtained from cinchona bark which is cultivated in the East Indies, India and Ceylon. In addition to its use in malaria it is also employed occasionally for other purposes in therapeutics. (See page 209.)

*Action in malaria.* When absorbed into the body, quinine and the other anti-malarial drugs circulate in the blood-stream, where they have the power of destroying malarial parasites, especially the young ones just discharged from a parent red corpuscle.

*Treatment of an attack.* Various régimes and dosage schemes are employed. The following is an example:

Quinine sulphate, 30 grains daily (i.e. o·6 gram, 10 grains, t.d.s.), by mouth for four consecutive days, followed by 1·2 gram (20 grains) daily two days a week (Saturdays and Sundays) for the next 8 weeks.

Subsequent anæmia may be treated with iron, and virulent types of the disease may need other measures.

### Other uses of quinine

1. *Antipyretic.* Quinine has an antipyretic action and is occasionally used in the treatment of coryza and mild febrile illnesses. Ammoniated tincture of quinine is a favourite preparation.

2. As a *bitter*. Quinine has a bitter flavour and helps to improve the appetite. It is therefore sometimes included in tonics.

3. In *obstetrics*. Its use for the medical induction of labour has been mentioned, page 209.

4. In *surgery*. Quinine and urethane solutions have been used for the injection of varicose veins.

Quinine and urea hydrochloride, 1 per cent, may be injected to produce local relief from pain in fibrositis, lumbago, etc.

### Some preparations of quinine

**Quinine sulphate** (*Quininæ sulphas*), 0·6 gram (1 to 10 grains).

This is also contained in ammoniated tincture or solution of quinine and in various quinine mixtures.

**Quinine bisulphate.      Quinine dihydrochloride.**

*Quinine poisoning and idiosyncrasy*, see page 29.

**Quinidine** (see page 91) is another alkaloid obtained from cinchona and is used in the treatment of auricular fibrillation.

## GOLD SALTS

Gold salts are used in therapeutics in the treatment of rheumatoid arthritis.

The first preparation to be employed was 'Sanocrysin' (gold sodium thiosulphate), for the treatment of pulmonary tuberculosis. The exact mode of action of gold salts in rheumatoid arthritis is uncertain.

A number of preparations are available, and are given by intramuscular injection. The one usually employed is injection of sodium aurothiomalate ('Myocrisin').

*Dosage.* The dosage varies according to the case. As a rule small doses at weekly intervals, commencing with 10 mg., increasing gradually up to 100 mg. are the maximum employed. Courses, therefore, last for some weeks, and after an interval of 2 months may be repeated.

### Toxic effects

Gold, when injected, has a cumulative effect owing to its slow excretion. Important toxic results may be observed, especially in some persons who show special idiosyncrasy and when large doses are used. They include:

Skin eruptions.

Stomatitis.

Diarrhœa.

Blood disorders, including agranulocytosis and purpura.

Albuminuria. It is wise to test the urine of all patients receiving gold at regular intervals.

It is also necessary to avoid exposure to direct sunlight by sun-bathing and also ultra-violet light while gold is being given, because permanent pigmentation of the skin may follow. Dimercaprol (B.A.L.) is used in the treatment of overdosage.

## ALCOHOL

The therapeutic use of alcoholic liquor has been steadily decreasing in medical practice, and although some physicians use it freely, others exclude it entirely. The true position is that it probably has a limited sphere of usefulness.

The opportunity of administering alcohol is often placed in the hands of the nurse, who should therefore have some knowledge of its value and danger. She will be wise, how-ever, never to give alcohol in any form unless it is prescribed by the doctor.

### The action of alcohol

Alcohol is frequently called a stimulant (and ordered in a "stimulant book"). This description is incorrect. The apparent stimulating action is actually the result of its de-pressing effect on the higher centres of the brain, whereby normal mental control and anxiety are removed to greater or less degree. Alcohol is not a cardiac stimulant, nor does it increase the activity of the respiratory centre. Its apparent effect on the circulation is due to the dilatation of the blood-vessels in the skin and the associated feeling of warmth, a property which may be of value in fainting attacks.

A similar action on the mucous membrane of the stomach produces a sensation of internal warmth which, in some cases, improves the appetite, an effect which can also be produced by suitable medicinal bitters.

It is oxidized in the tissues into carbon dioxide and water and is therefore to some extent of food value, especially as it is easily and quickly absorbed from the stomach.

Alcohol taken in large amounts and over a long period may have serious deleterious effects upon the body in certain individuals, producing such conditions as cirrhosis of the liver, chronic gastritis, peripheral neuritis or mental deterioration, but these effects need not be considered in connection with its medicinal administration.

## The uses of alcohol

When prescribed in acute disease it is generally given in the form of brandy or whisky, while in chronic conditions various wines, beer or stout may be employed.

It is not always wise to cut off completely its supply from a patient suffering from an acute disease who is accustomed to its use. On the other hand, there are few conditions in the young adult in which it is of any value.

In some cases of gastro-enteritis in infants, sherry-whey is useful, and in broncho-pneumonia in babies small doses of brandy often induce sleep and act as an easily absorbed foodstuff. Iced champagne occasionally is useful in cases of excessive vomiting in adults.

Alcohol is definitely contra-indicated in most of the acute fevers and, although formerly used a great deal in diphtheria, especially when cardiac complications were present, it has been shown to be quite useless and without effect in this condition.

The average case of pneumonia in an adult does not benefit from the use of alcohol, but in some instances, especially in the later stages and in the elderly, it may help to improve the general condition by acting as an easily absorbed foodstuff and by inducing sleep by its depressing effect on the nervous system.

In many diseases its use must be forbidden, especially gastric or duodenal ulcer, chronic gastritis and cirrhosis of the liver.

It must also be remembered that alcohol increases the action of barbiturates so that the two should never be taken together.

While its indiscriminate administration must be condemned, the use of alcohol is certainly justified if it produces a feeling of well-being (euphoria) in the terminal stages of pulmonary tuberculosis or in patients dying from inoperable cancer and similar conditions.

## External uses

It has already been mentioned (page 40) that alcohol and methylated spirit have antiseptic properties and that they harden the skin. Further, their rapid evaporation makes them a useful basis for cooling lotions in the treatment of sprains and contusions.

SUMMARY OF THE ACTION OF ALCOHOL

*Internal.*   A cerebral depressant.
             A vaso-dilator.
             An easily absorbed foodstuff.
*External.*   An antiseptic and disinfectant.
             Hardens the skin.
             Cooling effect due to rapid evaporation.

## Dangers of internal administration

(a) *Intoxication.* Loss of control of higher centres of the brain, leading to disorders of behaviour and unbalanced judgement.

Ataxia and speech disorders.

Coma (in large doses).

(b) *Chronic alcoholism.*

Habit formation.

Gastritis.

Neuritis.

Cirrhosis of the liver.

Mental deterioration.

Lowering of general resistance. This is shown by the seriousness of pneumonia in chronic alcoholics. They also tolerate general anæsthetics badly.

## The alcohol content of various wines and spirits, etc.

| | |
|---|---|
| Liqueurs - - - - | 50 per cent |
| Brandy, whisky, rum, gin - | 40 per cent |
| Port and sherry - - - | 20 per cent |
| Burgundy - - - up to | 14 per cent |
| Champagne, claret, hock - | 10 per cent |
| Beer and stout - - | 2 to 5 per cent |

# CHAPTER 16

# CHEMOTHERAPY AND THE SULPHONAMIDE DRUGS

For many years chemists and physicians have been working to produce chemical substances which would influence bacterial disease. An early outcome was the preparation of the arsenical compounds for use in the treatment of syphilis. Later it was found that certain complicated chemical compounds of the sulphonamide type, of which 'Prontosil' or Sulphanilamide was the first, were effective in the treatment of streptococcal infections. This led to the preparation of numerous other compounds of the same kind and their employment in other varieties of bacterial disease. Some years later the antibiotics were discovered.

Although sulphonamides have been superseded by antibiotics in the treatment of many diseases, they still play an important part in the management of some types of meningitis, bacillary dysentry and B. Coli infections of the urinary tract.

They may also be useful against organisms which have become resistant to antibiotics but have remained sensitive to sulphonamides, or may be given to patients who have developed sensitivity reactions to antibiotics.

## *Mode of action*

Sulphonamides do not actually kill bacteria but prevent their growth and multiplication in the body so that the natural immunity of the individual can exterminate the infection. They probably act by preventing bacteria from using para-amino-benzoic acid, a substance necessary in their metabolism. They are, therefore, bacteriostatic in action. The main principle in their administration is to produce rapidly a high concentration of the substance in the blood and to maintain this concentration for some days, until pyrexia and symptoms due to the disease have subsided. In order to reduce the risk of the patient developing drug sensitivity or agranulocytosis their administration should not usually be continued for more than ten days. Experience has shown which particular compounds are the most effective against each type of organism.

With the exception of the meningococcus, which does not become resistant, most other organisms which are initially sensitive to sulphonamides may become resistant. Sensitivity tests are, therefore, important.

## THE SULPHONAMIDES

The widespread use and manufacture of these drugs has resulted in a multiplicity of preparations and names. According to their practical use they fall into three main groups:

(*a*)  Sulphonamides used for general infections.
(*b*)  Sulphonamides used for urinary infections.
(*c*)  Sulphonamides used for intestinal infections.
(*d*)  Sulphonamides for local use.

Those used for general infections may also be employed for the other purposes mentioned.

### Sulphonamides for general infections

The most important are:

Sulphadimidine ('Sulphamezathine')
Sulphadiazine

Others include:

Sulphathiazole        Sulphamerazine
Sulphafurazole ('Gantrisin')

Trisulphonamide ('Sulphatriad'), a mixture of sulphadiazine, sulphathiazole and sulphamerazine.

Long-acting sulphonamides one dose of which is sufficient to cover twenty-four hours include sulphamethoxypyridazine ('Midicel', 'Lederkyn').

Sulfaphenazole ('Orisulf'), 500 mg. twice daily, is used in the treatment of chronic bronchitis and other respiratory infections.

Among the conditions in which sulphonamide therapy has been used with success are:

***Streptococcal infections.*** Infection by the streptococcus may produce many different manifestations of disease. In most instances, however, penicillin or one of the other antibiotics will be the drug of choice.

The following are common conditions due to streptococcal infection: puerperal sepsis, erysipelas, tonsillitis, cellulitis, otitis media, acute mastoiditis and streptococcal meningitis.

Scarlet fever is also due to a streptococcus, but sulphonamides have not proved effective in the acute disease, although they are of some value in the treatment of certain complications, such as otitis media.

*Meningococcal infections.* Sulphadiazine is especially effective in the treatment of meningococcal meningitis. Meningococci do not become resistant to the drug.

*Gonococcal infections.* Sulphonamides have been employed in the treatment of gonorrhœa both in the acute and chronic stages, but one of the antibiotics is usually employed.

*Pneumococcal infections.* Not every case of pneumonia responds and usually penicillin or one of the other antibiotics is employed.

## Sulphonamides for urinary infections

In addition to the sulphonamides mentioned above for use in general infections, the following are particularly active against the Bacillus Coli and are, therefore, employed in cases of pyelitis and cystitis:

Sulphamethizole ('Urolucosil', 100-200 mg.)
Sulphacetamide ('Albucid')

## Sulphonamides for intestinal infections

All the sulphonamides previously mentioned are soluble and are, therefore, easily absorbed into the blood stream from the alimentary tract. There are a number of insoluble sulphonamides which are not absorbed and therefore continue to act on bacteria throughout in the whole length of the bowel. This local action is of great advantage in the treatment of bacillary dysentery and other intestinal infections in which a general effect is not required. There is less risk of urinary crystallization in these conditions in which much fluid may be lost from the body by diarrhoea.

Sulphaguanidine
Phthalylsulphathiazole ('Sulfathalidine')
Succinylsulphathiazole ('Sulfasuxidine', 'Cremosuxidine')
Phthalyl sulphacetamide ('Enterocid')

Salicylazosulphapyridine ('Salazopyrin') is a sulphonamide used in the treatment of ulcerative colitis.

Being insoluble considerably larger doses than those of the other sulphonamides are used.

## Sulphonamides for local use

Sulphonamides are occasionally applied to the skin in the form of ointments in the treatment of various skin diseases, but it must be remembered that they may cause sensitization and dermatitis and are, therefore, best avoided. In powder form (sometimes combined with penicillin) they may be applied to ulcers or open wounds.

Sulphacetamide eye drops and eye ointment are however, very useful in the treatment of infections of the conjunctiva.

### Methods of administration

In the majority of cases the drugs are given by mouth but, to gravely ill patients and those who vomit excessively, sodium salt preparations may be administered by intramuscular injection or intravenously. They may be conveniently given by the latter method when the patient is receiving saline by the continuous intravenous drip technique by injecting the required dose at regular intervals through the rubber tubing leading to the vein.

### Dosage

When given for general infections the dosage of the soluble sulphonamides must be carefully adjusted to the age of the patient. It is usual to commence with a single large dose (double that which is subsequently given) in order to ensure a rapid high concentration of the drug in the blood. Tablets of the drug (each of which usually contains 0·5 gram) are given by mouth and may be chewed or powdered and swallowed with a glass of water. An alternative and better method is to crush and suspend in milk, glucose saline or a mucilage of tragacanth. If the drug is not tolerated by mouth, special preparations for intramuscular injection may be used. It must be emphasized, however, that deep intramuscular injections must be given into the buttock. Subcutaneous injection leads to the gradual formation of a painful abscess, leaving an ulcer which takes a long time to heal.

The usual initial adult dose is 2 grams, followed by 1 gram four-hourly. (Sulphadiazine is given every 6 to 8 hours and 'Sulphamerazine' every 8 to 12 hours.) The administration of the drug is generally continued for a day or two after the temperature has fallen to normal, as premature withdrawal is often followed by recurrence of pyrexia and the infective process.

*Urinary infections.* Since the soluble sulphonamides are concentrated and excreted in the urine, smaller doses than those employed for general infections are required, e.g. Trisulphonamide ('Sulphatriad') 0·5 gram every four to six hours, Sulphamethizole ('Urolucosil') 100-200 mg. every four hours.

N.B.—Long-acting sulphonamides are given once or twice daily.

*For infants the following is useful:*

| Age - - - | 1-3 months | 6 months | 3 years | 5 years |
|---|---|---|---|---|
| Daily dose in grams (approx.) - - | 1 | 1½ | 2½ | 3 |

The main principles to be observed in the administration of sulphonamide drugs are:

1. They should only be used against susceptible organisms.

2. An adequate fluid intake with a correspondingly appropriate urinary output should be maintained, viz.:

Not less than 3 to 4 pints intake.

Not less than 1½ to 2 pints output.

It is a wise precaution to record these measurements as a routine. At the same time it is desirable to render the urine alkaline with potassium citrate.

3. Adequate dosage must be given so that a constant and effective blood concentration is maintained.

4. The administration should not be prolonged for more than 5 to 7 days except in special cases when control blood counts should be taken.

## Complications of sulphonamide therapy

As in the case of other valuable drugs, the sulphonamides not only bring their benefits but also their dangers. It is natural that there should be a tendency to use such valuable remedies on every possible occasion and, although considerable latitude is permissible, their employment should be tempered with discretion and it must be remembered that patients taking them often feel quite as ill from their effects as they do from the original infection.

1. *Minor toxic effects.* These are common and include nausea, vomiting, headache, general lassitude, mental depression and sometimes pyrexia ("drug fever") which continues after that due to the original infection has subsided. These symptoms rapidly vanish when the drug has been withdrawn.

For vomiting, tincture of opium, 5 minims half an hour before each dose, or phenobarbitone may be tried. If severe, and the continuation of the drug is essential, tablets by mouth are replaced by intramuscular injections.

2. *Hæmaturia.* Crystals of sulphapyridine, sulphathiazole and sulphadiazine compounds can often be seen in the urine as a hazy cloud in patients taking full doses of the drugs. In some instances these crystals affect the tubules of the kidneys and produce blood in the urine complete blockage of the tubules will lead to anæmia and uræmia which might prove fatal. This is most likely to occur when the urine is concentrated and the patient is not taking sufficient fluid or is suffering from diarrhœa or severe sweating. The treatment consists of stopping the drug and giving potassium citrate and additional fluids by mouth. This is a most important complication for the nurse to observe.

3. *Anæmia.* Some cases develop severe anæmia, especially after prolonged dosage, which is treated with iron.

4. *Agranulocytosis.* This is fortunately a less common but very serious complication which may prove fatal. Most cases appear to be due to overdosage, but some are due to idiosyncrasy after quite moderate amounts. White cell counts are, therefore, advisable when large doses are given.

5. *Cyanosis.* A bluish tinge of the skin and mucous membranes is quite commonly produced by sulphanilamide and sulphapyridine but is rarely observed when other sulphonamides are used. It is due to the drug causing certain changes in the hæmoglobin in the blood (the formation of sulphæmoglobin and methæmoglobin).

6. Occasionally skin eruptions and neuritis may develop.

# CHAPTER 17

# ANTIBIOTICS

An antibiotic is a chemical substance produced by micro-organisms or moulds which prevents the growth (bacteriostatic) of or kills (bactericidal) other micro-organisms.

The most important are:

Penicillin.

The Tetracycline group

(a) Tetracycline ('Tetracyn').

(b) Chlortetracycline ('Aureomycin').

(c) Oxytetracycline ('Terramycin').

Erythromycin, Novobiocin, Spiramycin, Oleandomycin.

Chloramphenicol ('Chloromycetin').

Polymyxin B and Bacitracin.

Nystatin, Griseofulvin.

Streptomycin, Viomycin.

Each antibiotic has its own sphere of activity against the common bacteria. Some are effective against a wide range of organisms, to others only a few are sensitive, but fortunately most of the common organisms are affected by at least one of the antibiotics. On the other hand, the only viruses which are sensitive are those causing virus pneumonia and psittacosis, which are sensitive to the tetracycline group. Unfortunately, the other more common viruses, causing poliomyelitis, measles, mumps, chicken-pox and small-pox are uninfluenced by any of the present known antibiotics.

## Disadvantages

### (1) Bacterial resistance.

As with sulphonamides, an important drawback to the use of antibiotics is that many bacteria acquire resistance to them after a period of treatment and continue to breed resistant organisms which can cause further disease. This will no longer respond to treatment with the same antibiotic. For example, the tubercle bacillus quickly develops resistance to streptomycin. Staphylococci also acquire resistance both to penicillin and drugs of the tetracycline group.

## (2) Toxic effects and sensitivity

Gastro-intestinal irritation, nausea, vomiting and diarrhœa may occur when antibiotics are given by mouth.

Skin sensitivity may develop to penicillin or streptomycin causing rashes, not only in patients but also in nurses and others handling the drug. Streptomycin may have a serious toxic effect on the vestibular and auditory nerve causing vertigo and deafness.

Very rarely anaphylactic shock with collapse and even death may follow the administration of penicillin in hypersensitive individuals.

In hospital patients, for future reference, it is wise to make a conspicuous note on their records if *any* drug sensitivity is observed.

## (3) Super-infection.

This applies especially to the antibiotics given by mouth which by killing off some of the normal bacteria inhabiting the alimentary canal permit the overgrowth of other insensitive ones which can cause serious complications.

In particular, there may be an overgrowth of yeasts and fungi (usually Monilia Albicans, the fungus causing thrush) which cause soreness of the mouth and anal regions, or which may even extend into the bronchi and lungs with fatal results.

Staphylococci may develop resistance to penicillin and the tetracyclines and cause serious gastro-enteritis or other infections. The only antibiotics, to which such resistant staphylococci are likely to be susceptible are Erythromycin, Chloramphenicol, Novobiocin, Neomycin, or Oleandomycin.

(4) Alterations in vitamin formation and absorption from the bowel. Vitamin B, including riboflavin and nicotinic acid, is particularly affected, so that this is sometimes given at the same time as an oral antibiotic, although this is probably only necessary if the administration is prolonged beyond five days and in debilitated patients.

(5) In susceptible individuals chloramphenicol may occasionally produce aplastic anæmia or agranulocytosis.

## Penicillin

This substance, which was the first antibiotic to be used, is the active principle of a mould (*Penicillium notaιum*) which has a marked action on many bacteria. In average doses it is bacteriostatic but if high blood levels are produced it may be bactericidal. In many instances it is even more effective than the sulphonamide drugs and has practically no toxic effects except in sensitive individuals. Although it has a wide range of action not all bacteria are affected by it and even some of those which are can eventually develop some degree of resistance to it.

It may be given by intramuscular injection or intravenously, and may also be applied locally to septic areas.

In addition to the natural substance, synthetic penicillins can be prepared. Their chemical structure can, therefore, be varied and may be of value when bacterial resistance has developed, e.g. Methicillin ('Celbenin').

### Indications

The suitability of a case for treatment with penicillin depends not so much on the nature of the disease as on the susceptibility of the micro-organism causing it: some species are highly susceptible and others far too resistant for this treatment to have any effect. It follows that in diseases which may be caused by any of several different bacteria (e.g. meningitis, peritonitis) a bacteriological diagnosis and sensitivity test is usually necessary if treatment is to be undertaken with any assurance of success.

The chief organisms susceptible to penicillin are:

| | |
|---|---|
| Gonococcus | Diphtheria bacillus |
| Meningococcus | Organisms of gas-gangrene |
| Streptococcus | Spirochaetes of syphilis: possibly of |
| Staphylococcus | Weil's disease |
| Pneumococcus | Actinomyces |
| Influenza bacillus( ?) | Anthrax bacillus |

Examples of *diseases in which penicillin may be used* are:

| | | |
|---|---|---|
| septicæmia | actinomycosis | carbuncles |
| puerperal sepsis | anthrax | suppurative arthritis |
| cellulitis | gonorrhœa | malignant endocarditis |
| osteomyelitis | gas gangrene | syphilis |
| pneumonia | meningitis | |

*Penicillin is of no value* in the following conditions for which it should *not* be used except when some intercurrent infection is present:

(a) Tuberculosis      (c) Rheumatoid arthritis

(b) Acute rheumatic fever      (d) Ulcerative colitis

(e) Infections caused by viruses such as influenza, poliomyelitis and encephalitis.

(f) All gram negative bacillary infections such as whooping cough, typhoid fever, dysentery, undulant fever, and infections with Bacillus coli.

(g) Glandular fever      (j) Leukæmia

(h) Pemphigus      (k) Malaria

(i) Hodgkin's disease      (l) Cancer

## Administration

Unless the following properties of penicillin are appreciated, unsatisfactory therapeutic results are likely to be obtained.

(a) Once penicillin has been removed from the ampoule or tube it is likely to deteriorate, particularly if exposed to moisture or heat. Solutions or other preparations of penicillin exposed to air and kept at room temperature will not deteriorate significantly in 24 hours, but should be kept in a refrigerator.

(b) Penicillin is rapidly destroyed by boiling, by most antiseptics, and by many of the common air bacteria.

(c) Only special preparations can be given effectively by mouth e.g. penicillin V and some synthetic forms e.g. 'Broxil', 'Falapen'.

(d) Penicillin passes rapidly from the blood into the tissues, but the serous membranes and meninges present a barrier which penicillin does not readily penetrate. Hence intrathecal and intrapleural injections may be necessary.

(e) Penicillin is rapidly excreted; for this reason it must be given in sufficient dosage to maintain an adequate concentration in the blood.

(*f*) The diffusion of penicillin into dead tissues is slow; sequestra, large sloughs, or collections of pus, are, therefore, likely to harbour bacteria out of reach of the drug, and these usually have to be removed if treatment is to be effective.

## Types of Penicillin

Penicillin is an acid substance which forms salts with sodium, potassium and calcium and can be combined with other substances.

There are therefore several different forms of penicillin which differ somewhat from each other and are used for special purposes.

1. **Benzyl penicillin** or **soluble penicillin** (known also as crystalline penicillin G) which is commonly employed for repeated intramuscular injections. 'Falapen' is a form of benzyl penicillin which may be administered orally in twice daily doses of 500,000 units, preferably before a meal.

2. **Procaine penicillin,** sometimes prescribed as 'Distaquaine,' which is less soluble and therefore more slowly absorbed. It is given in doses of 300,000-600,000 units daily by intramuscular injection. In order to get a more rapid effect the first injection may be combined with a similar dose of soluble benzyl penicillin.

3. **Benzathine penicillin** ('Penidural') and benethamine penicillin ('Benapen') which are even less soluble and more slowly absorbed. A single intramuscular injection of 600,000-1 million units may give an effective blood level lasting several days. A hard lump may develop at the site of injection.

4. **Phenoxymethyl penicillin.** (Penicillin V) is used for oral administration. It is not destroyed, like benzyl penicillin, by the acid of the stomach. It is given in doses of 250 mg. every four to six hours.

5. Combinations of the various types of penicillin are available. Oily preparations which delay absorption are sometimes used (e.g. Procaine penicillin in oil with aluminium monostearate, P.A.M.) and there are other preparations in

which penicillin is mixed with streptomycin (e.g. 'Crystamycin' or sulphonamides.

N.B.—Penicillin is not usually administered at the same time as tetracycline.

### Systematic administration

Penicillin may be administered in the following ways:

(1) *Intramuscular injection* of 500,000 to 1,000,000 units of soluble (benzyl) penicillin is given every six to eight hours or twice daily, according to the severity of the infection. Procaine penicillin ('Distaquaine') is given in doses of 300,000 to 600,000 units once daily.

N.B.—One million units is sometimes called one Mega unit.

(2) *Intravenous injection.* Soluble penicillin may be injected intravenously in doses similar to those given by intramuscular injection depending on the nature and severity of the infection.

(3) *Intrathecal injection* may be used in certain cases of meningitis. Only specially prepared soluble (benzyl) penicillin well diluted, should be employed. One dose of 20,000 units in twenty four hours is sufficient.

(4) *Intrapleural injection* may be used in the treatment of empyema.

(5) *Local application.* Penicillin may be used either in the form of a solution, a cream or a powder. In the latter instance it may be mixed with a sulphonamide and blown with an insufflator onto raw surfaces or into wounds twice daily. Solutions may be used for the irrigation of wounds or sinuses and as eye drops, ear drops and nasal drops. Creams may be applied daily for lesions on the surface of the body.

Apart from eye drops, local applications are inadvisable and should be discouraged on account of the liability of producing a sensitization rash which may be worse than the original condition.

(6) *Oral penicillin.* Special preparations are particularly useful for children but may also be effective in adults if the infection is not too severe.

*The duration of treatment* varies considerably according to the condition and response of the patient, but should seldom be for less than 5 days or more than 12 days. Treatment is usually continued for about 2 days after a favourable response has been obtained. If no response is obtained within 72 hours another antibiotic will probably be needed.

*The dosage* described above is recommended for all conditions requiring systemic treatment except the following:

1. Syphilis: In the early stages a single large dose of procaine penicillin in oil (P.A.M.), e.g. 2·4 million units (or 4 c.c. into each buttock) followed by 600,000 units daily for 10 days is probably sufficient. In the later stages smaller doses may be effective. 1 million units of soluble penicillin in divided doses daily may also be used.

2. Gonorrhœa: in uncomplicated cases a single dose of procaine penicillin in oil (P.A.M.), 300,000 units is usually effective.

3. Bacterial endocarditis: a daily dose of 1 to 5 million units is necessary for at least a month, but even prolonged treatment may be unsuccessful.

4. Actinomycosis: the dosage varies considerably according to the sensitivity of the actinomyces.

*Toxic reactions.* Penicillin is usually non-toxic, but it occasionally gives rise to minor reactions, such as fever, and urticarial rashes. These may be treated with antihistamine drugs and the local application of Calamine lotion.

Rarely, as previously mentioned, anaphylactic shock with collapse and even death may occur. In this type of reaction adrenaline 1 ml. (1 in 1000) should be injected subcutaneously at once, followed by an intravenous antihistamine (e.g. 'Benadryl') and, if necessary by intravenous hydrocortisone. Before giving penicillin, therefore, it is wise to enquire about previous sensitivity and also if the patient is subject to asthma or other allergic conditions.

## Chloramphenicol ('Chloromycetin')

This is a crystalline substance obtained from the mould

*Streptomyces Venezuelæ* and which can also be prepared synthetically.

It is particularly valuable in the treatment of typhoid fever which is not materially affected by any other antibiotic. Also in meningitis caused by *H. Influenzae*.

Although it may also be used in virus pneumonia, some staphylococcal infections, whooping cough, infections of the urinary tract, gonorrhœa and undulant fever, one of the other antibiotics is generally safer unless the organism is insensitive to them.

This is because some individuals, especially children, are sensitive to chloramphenicol and the drug may affect the bone marrow causing aplastic anæmia or agranulocytosis which may prove fatal. There is no way of anticipating this and it may occur after relatively small doses. The danger to adults is very small provided the course of treatment does not exceed ten days.

It is supplied in capsules each containing 0·25 gram. It has a bitter taste which is sometimes a disadvantage when given to children unless concealed in honey or given in the form of a special preparation ('Chloromycetin palmitate').

The average daily dose is 50 to 75 mg. per kilogram body weight or 0·5 gram every four or six hours.

Ointments are available, also eye drops and ear drops. These local applications are free from the danger of producing agranulocytosis.

### The Tetracycline group of antibiotics

These include:

(*a*) **tetracycline** ('Tetracyn', 'Achromycin', 'Ambramycin').

(*b*) **chlortetracycline** ('Aureomycin').

(*c*) **oxytetracycline** ('Terramycin').

Although 'Aureomycin' and 'Terramycin' were the first drugs of this group to be isolated and used, chemically they are both derived from a substance tetracycline which also has antibiotic effects similar to both of the others.

'Aureomycin' and 'Terramycin' differ slightly in chemical composition but have a very similar antibiotic range which covers not only those organisms which are generally sensitive to penicillin but also the virus causing virus pneumonia and a number of other organisms. They are particularly useful against staphylococci which are resistant to penicillin, but it must be remembered that staphylococci can also develop resistance against them.

They are usually given by mouth in doses of 0·5 gram followed by 0·25 gram every 4 to 6 hours for four to five days.

Special preparations are available for intravenous and intramuscular injections and local applications such as drops and ointments are also in use.

### Erythromycin (200-500 mg., 6 hourly)

This is another antibiotic having a similar range of action. Its main use is against staphylococci which have become resistant to all other antibiotics. Resistance to Erythromycin also develops rapidly so that its use should be restricted to selected and urgent cases. Proprietary preparations include 'Erythrocin' and 'Ilotycin'. Intravenous injections are available.

**Novobiocin.** ('Albamycin', 'Cathomycin') is particularly useful against staphylococcal infections which are resistant to other antibiotics.

**Spiramycin, Oleandomycin.** ('Matromycin', 'Romicil', 'Sigmamycin' which also contains tetracycline. All the above have properties and uses similar to Erythromycin.

### Special Antibiotics

There are a number of antibiotics which are occasionally used for special purposes. They tend to be toxic and are therefore limited in their application. They include:

**Neomycin** is of value in some gastro-intestinal infections and may also be applied locally to the skin.

**Bacitracin,** an antibiotic derived from bacillus subtilis which has a limited use against streptococci, staphylococci and some other organisms. It may have a toxic effect on the kidneys and is only given by injection in selected cases when other antibiotics have failed (dose 20,000 units, 6 hourly). It may safely be applied locally to infected wounds.

**Polymyxin** (including Aerosporin) is effective against

Bacillus pyocyaneus and certain other uncommon organisms. It is given in doses of 250,000 units every four to six hours by intramuscular injection. It can be given intrathecally in special cases of meningitis.

**Tyrothricin and Gramicidin** may be used as local applications.

**Nystatin.** This is a special antibiotic which has no action on ordinary bacteria but is effective against fungi and yeasts such as Monilia albicans. It may be applied locally for thrush and pessaries are available for vaginal infections. Doses of 500,000 to 1 million units may be given by mouth for intestinal and general monilia infections especially those following administration of tetracycline.

**Griseofulvin** is used in the treatment of fungus infections of the skin, including ringworm. The usual dose is 1 G. daily. Treatment may be prolonged if the nails are affected.

## Streptomycin

This is an antibiotic obtained from a soil organism called *Actinomyces Griseus*. It is interesting to note that in the process of its manufacture Vitamin $B_{12}$ is formed, a fact which has made the preparation of the latter substance commercially possible.

Although streptomycin is used mainly in the treatment of tuberculosis, it is also active against a number of organisms (especially gram negative bacilli, many of which are insensitive to penicillin, e.g. *Bacillus Coli*), which accounts for its usefulness in a number of other conditions. These include some types of pneumonia, peritonitis, cholecystitis, infection of the urinary tract and any condition caused by organisms which are shown by bacteriological test to be insensitive to penicillin or the other antibiotics. In these conditions its administration is only continued for a few days. Streptomycin may be combined with penicillin for use in some infections.

Like other antibiotics it has certain *disadvantages* which include:

1. Not only the tubercle bacillus but also other organisms rapidly acquire a tolerance to it and permanently resistant

strains of micro-organisms are produced which will no longer respond to treatment with it.

2. If prolonged or heavy dosage, which may sometimes appear necessary in tuberculosis, is employed there is a risk of causing serious toxic effects which include damage to the eighth cranial nerve and the symptoms of deafness, giddiness and tinnitus. These symptoms may gradually clear up but in some cases are permanent.

3. Persons who handle the drug may become sensitive to it after a few weeks and may develop a dermatitis of the hands, forearm and around the eyes, which is often very intractable to treatment. Rubber gloves should, therefore, always be worn when administering streptomycin.

Streptomycin is used in the treatment of all forms of tuberculosis, the dosage and duration of treatment depends on the individual case.

In pulmonary tuberculosis the dose does not usually exceed 1·0 gram daily for thirty days.

In tuberculous meningitis, intrathecal injections of 0·1 gram in 5 to 10 c.c. of distilled water may be given in addition to intramuscular injections.

It is not absorbed when given by mouth but may be given in this way in certain intestinal infections.

## Para-amino salicylic acid (P.A.S.)

This drug which is usually prescribed in the form of its sodium salt (**Sodium aminosalicylate**), is not an antibiotic in the ordinary sense but it is used in conjunction with streptomycin for two reasons:

(1) It has itself an action on the tubercle bacillus.

(2) It delays the development of streptomycin resistance.

The usual dose is 12 grams daily (4G t.d.s.) for periods of up to three months.

It has a bitter taste and may be taken in water with or without flavouring agents, or in cachets.

In some cases the urine of patients taking P.A.S. reduces Benedict's reagent. It may cause nausea, vomiting and diarrhœa.

**Isoniazid,** isonicotinic acid hydrazide (**I.N.A.H.**) 'Nidrazid', 'Pycazide', 'Rimifon' etc.

This is a synthetic substance which has a similar action and which may be given with streptomycin.

The average dose is 200 mg. of isoniazid daily in divided doses.

It passes through the meninges into the cerebrospinal fluid and given with streptomycin, is of importance in the treatment of tuberculous meningitis.

*'Inapasade'* granules contain both P.A.S. and I.N.H. and are a convenient form of administration. The average dose is 2 scoopsful twice daily.

Because the tubercle bacillus quickly develops resistance to streptomycin, sodium aminosalicylate and isoniazid when they are given separately (but this is delayed when combinations are used), it is usual to give two of the drugs together, e.g.

(1) Streptomycin 1 gram with isoniazid 200 mg. daily.
(2) Streptomycin 1 gram with sodium aminosalicylate 12 grams daily.
(3) Streptomycin 1 gram twice or thrice weekly with sodium aminosalicylate 12 grams daily.
(4) Sometimes Isoniazid and sodium aminosalicylate are given together without streptomycin.

Each course may be continued for several months.

**Viomycin** may be used against tubercle bacilli which have become resistant to streptomycin but it tends to produce severe toxic effects and must not be given to patients with impairment of renal function.

**Cycloserine** is an oral antibiotic, the dose of which should not exceed 1 G. daily. Its use is similar to viomycin. Both these drugs may be combined with isoniazid or P.A.S.

# CHAPTER 18

# VACCINES, SERA AND OTHER BIOLOGICAL PRODUCTS

The preparation and use of vaccines and sera are closely connected with the subject of immunity. By ***immunity*** is meant the ability of an individual to resist disease, and it is dependent on:

   (i) the power of the leucocytes to destroy bacteria,

   (ii) the presence of antibodies in the tissues which kill bacteria or of antitoxins which neutralize their toxins.

Immunity may be:

1. Natural or inborn.

2. Acquired:

    (*a*) As a result of recovery from infection.

    (*b*) Artificially produced.

        (i) Active immunity (e.g. by the use of vaccines and toxoids).

        (ii) Passive immunity (by the use of serum).

## Vaccines

Strictly speaking, a vaccine is a suspension of germs which have been killed. It therefore contains the toxins of the organisms, but because the germs are no longer alive and cannot multiply, they do not cause the actual disease in the body. The toxins, however, have the power to stimulate the production of antibodies and, in this way, to raise the resistance of the individual to the particular organism causing the disease.

The vaccine lymph used in the prevention of small-pox differs from other vaccines since it contains the living organisms which cause cow-pox or vaccinia. The immunity produced by its use depends on the fact that the individual vaccinated contracts cow-pox, which is a local lesion at the site of the inoculation. The antibodies to cow-pox are apparently the same as those to small-pox and therefore an immunity to small-pox remains after the local lesion has healed

In addition to the above types of vaccine, preparations are sometimes made of the toxins alone, without the dead bodies of the bacteria.

The production of immunity by vaccines is called "active" because the tissues of the individual are stimulated to produce antibodies for themselves.

Bacterial vaccines may be either:

(a) *Autogenous*, that is, prepared from cultures of germs obtained from the patient to be treated.

(b) *Stock vaccines*, made from cultures of the organism kept in the laboratory.

## Technique

The skin at the site selected for the injection, usually the upper arm close to the insertion of the deltoid muscle, is cleansed with ether or tincture of iodine and the required dose injected subcutaneously with a fine needle. In the majority of instances, injections are repeated at intervals of not less than a week.

## Reactions

The administration of a vaccine is frequently followed by a reaction which may be either local or general.

(a) Local reactions, with pain, swelling and redness at the site of injection may appear in 12 to 24 hours.

(b) General reactions. These include a rise in temperature and, sometimes, an increase in the symptoms of the disease for which the vaccine is given. The temperature should, therefore, be charted four-hourly after the injection of a vaccine.

## Uses

Vaccines may be used either in the treatment or the prevention of a disease.

## Therapeutic uses of vaccines

Vaccines are sometimes used in the treatment of the following diseases:

Acne.
Staphylococcal infections (e.g. boils).

## Prophylactic uses

The following vaccines are used to produce an immunity which will prevent the individual from contracting the disease, or modify its severity, if the patient subsequently happens to come in contact with the organism concerned. The immunity produced lasts from one to several years. "Boosting" doses are therefore, usually necessary.

## Typhoid vaccine

The vaccine generally employed to produce immunity to enteric fever contains killed typhoid bacilli together with the bacilli which cause paratyphoid A and paratyphoid B, in order that it may be effective against all the organisms of the typhoid group. It is sometimes called T.A.B., and usually contains:

| | |
|---|---|
| Typhoid bacilli | 1000 million. |
| Paratyphoid A | 500 million. |
| Paratyphoid B | 500 million. |

in 0·5 ml. which is the first dose given. A second dose of 1 ml. follows after an interval of ten days to three weeks. Those frequently exposed to infection should be revaccinated every six to twelve months.

A local reaction occurring at the site of injection, consisting of tenderness, redness and swelling after four hours is common. General symptoms including pyrexia or malaise lasting twenty four hours are quite common. The subject should therefore restrict activity during this period and avoid alcohol.

A preparation of the toxin of tetanus (tetanus toxoid) may be included in order to produce immunity to tetanus at the same time (T.A.B.T.). The interval between doses should be six weeks. A third dose may be given after six months.

## Poliomyelitis Vaccine

Specially prepared vaccines containing three types of poliomyelitis virus are available.

Dose: 1 ml. by intramuscular injection into the upper arm, repeated in three weeks and after seven months.

Neither local nor general reactions are to be expected but other vaccines, e.g. smallpox, yellow fever, B.C.G., should not be given within three to four weeks.

An oral vaccine is also in use. (Three doses of three drops on a piece of sugar at intervals of 4 to 6 weeks.)

## Anti-catarrh vaccines

These contain a mixture of the organisms associated with the common cold, including streptococci, staphylococci, pneumococci, influenza, bacilli and micrococcus catarrhalis. In order to be effective, a course of this vaccine is given early in the autumn before the "cold" season commences.

**Whooping-cough vaccines,** containing the Bordet-Gengou bacillus, are given in infancy and produce some degree of immunity to the disease. They are sometimes combined with diphtheria and tetanus prophylactics.

**Rabies, cholera, yellow fever** and **plague vaccines** are also prepared.

## Small-pox vaccination

The vaccine used for the prevention of small-pox is not a suspension of dead organisms in saline but lymph obtained from a calf containing the living virus of cow-pox.

*Vaccinia* is an acute infectious disease affecting cows and characterized by a pustular eruption which is confined to the udder and teats. It is believed that the condition is due to the infection by the organism of small-pox, the virulence of which is so modified by its passage through the body of the cow that only a localized lesion results.

It was found that human beings who contracted cow-pox as the result of milking infected cows remained immune to small-pox. Edward Jenner, in 1780, made use of this fact and commenced the practice of deliberate vaccination with vaccinia as a prevention against small-pox.

## Vaccination

The material used for purposes of vaccination is prepared in the following way. A healthy calf is inoculated with the virus of vaccinia. Vesicles of cow-pox develop on the udder of the calf. The lymph from these vesicles is then collected and mixed with glycerin, which acts as a preservative and kills any other germs which may be present. The final product, after tests have been employed to ensure its sterility, is placed in small glass tubes and is known as *glycerinated calf lymph.*

The usual technique of vaccination is as follows:

1. The site chosen for inoculation is cleaned with soap and water, followed if necessary by ether. Vaccination is usually performed on the upper and outer part of the left arm. The thigh or calf is sometimes selected for cosmetic reasons.

2. By means of a rubber bulb the lymph is blown out of its container on to the skin in one or more places. Originally, three or four separate inoculations were made, but at the present time one is generally considered to be sufficient except when an epidemic of severe oriental small-pox is prevalent.

3. Multiple pressure technique, using a triangular pointed (cutting) needle which is held almost parallel to the skin, fifteen to thirty applications of firm pressure are made through the drop of lymph. This is just sufficient to roughen the skin without drawing blood. The lymph is allowed to dry for five minutes and the area is covered with a square of lint or gauze which is kept in position by tapes or strapping.

4. Using a needle or the point of a scalpel, a scratch, half an inch long and not sufficiently deep to draw blood, is made in the skin. The lymph is rubbed in with the instrument and allowed to dry.

The following sequence of events takes place at the site of inoculation. On the third day a red papule appears, by the sixth day it has become a vesicle which reaches its maximum development on the eighth day and has a central (umbilicated) depression. By the tenth day a pustule is formed, with some surrounding redness and tenderness of the skin. The axillary glands may be painful. Slight fever and general malaise are often present. In the course of two or three days the pustule dries up leaving a scab which separates at the end of three weeks.

*After treatment.* It is essential to keep the vaccinated area dry, and for this reason it should not be immersed while bathing. Frequent changing of the dressing is undesirable and, provided it remains in place, need not be touched for the first ten days.

If the arm is painful it may be necessary to obtain rest and support by means of a sling. Care should be taken that the lesion is not accidentally injured.

*Complications.* (a) *Local sepsis,* which should not occur if the subject is in a good state of health and proper cleanliness is observed.

(b) Inflammation of the brain, or *post-vaccinal encephalitis* occasionally develops in children who are vaccinated for the first time between the ages of 3 and 13. This is a very fatal condition (mortality 30-40 per cent).

The law no longer demands that vaccination shall be performed on infants before the age of 6 months. In view of the possibility of post-vaccinal encephalitis in older children it is, however, advisable that all infants should be vaccinated.

The immunity conferred by vaccination lasts about three years and therefore revaccination should be performed at intervals of this duration in individuals who are likely to come in contact with the disease. A lesser degree of immunity persists for about seven years.

Recent successful vaccination produces complete immunity to small-pox, which develops in nine days from the time of inoculation. The incubation period of small-pox is approximately fourteen days. It follows, therefore, that an individual vaccinated within three or four days of exposure to small-pox will obtain protection.

### Tuberculosis vaccines

A preparation known as B.C.G. vaccine (Bacille Calmette-Guérin) and consisting of live tubercle bacilli specially cultured so that they have become non-virulent and unable to cause disease, has been used to produce immunity to tuberculosis in new-born infants of tuberculous parents and those who work in contact with tuberculosis, e.g. nurses who are found to be Mantoux negative. An intradermal dose of o·1 ml. produces a small papule which persists for some weeks. The Mantoux test should subsequently become positive.

## Bacterial toxins

In some instances, preparations are made from the toxins of bacteria and these are used to produce immunity in the same way as ordinary vaccines. In others, the actual toxins are much too poisonous for use and substances called *toxoids*, obtained from them by special chemical processes, are employed. A toxoid has the same immunizing properties as a toxin without its dangers.

In other instances, the toxin or toxoid may be mixed with an equivalent amount of antitoxin, which does not interfere with its immunizing power, to produce toxin- or toxoid-antitoxin mixtures.

### Diphtheria prophylactics

Various preparations of the above type have been employed to produce immunity to diphtheria, including:

Alum precipitated toxin (A.P.T.).

Diphtheria toxoid-antitoxin floccules (T.A.F.).

Formol toxoid (F.T.).

One or more doses at intervals of 3 to 4 weeks, depending on the preparation used, are given by subcutaneous injection.

**Tetanus Vaccine (Toxoid).** o·5 ml. is given by intramuscular injection followed by 1 ml. in six weeks. A further dose is advisable after six to eighteen months.

**Mixed vaccines.** Whooping cough vaccine may be combined with a tetanus and diphtheria prophylactic, three injections being given at intervals of one month. These inoculations are not usually given during an epidemic of poliomyelitis because they appear to increase the risk of acquiring this disease.

## Tests of immunity

Although bacterial toxins themselves are too dangerous for therapeutic use, very dilute solutions are used in order to test the immunity of individuals to certain diseases.

If a minute dose of toxin is injected into the skin (intradermally) and the individual has antibodies to that disease circulating in the blood, the effect of the toxin will be neutralized and there will be no reaction (negative response).

On the other hand, if the blood is deficient in antibodies, the toxin will produce local inflammation (redness, swelling, etc.) and the reaction is said to be positive. In other words, it indicates that the individual is susceptible to the disease. Examples of this are:

1. **The Schick test** for diphtheria.

A minute dose (0·2 ml.) of diluted diphtheria toxin is injected directly into the skin of the forearm (intradermally). If the individual has a sufficient amount of diphtheria anti-toxin circulating in the blood, the toxin is neutralized and no reaction takes place.

Such a patient is immune to diphtheria and the test is said to be negative.

On the other hand, if the patient has not sufficient antibodies to diphtheria present, an area of redness $\frac{1}{2}$ to 1 inch in diameter develops at the site of injection within twenty-four hours and persists for two to three days. This is a positive reaction.

A control injection is made into the other forearm consisting of diphtheria toxin which has been destroyed by heat. This is done in order to make sure that a positive reaction is due to the toxin and not to the protein contained in it, as some individuals are sensitive to the protein alone.

*Immunization.* Those patients who have been found to be susceptible to diphtheria by means of the Schick test can be rendered immune by injecting one of the diphtheria prophylactics already mentioned. The body is stimulated to produce a supply of antibodies which lasts for several years. Two or more subcutaneous injections are given and immunity develops about six weeks after the last injection has been made. By this means it has been found possible to reduce very considerably the incidence of infection among school children and among those nursing diphtheria.

2. **The Dick test** for scarlet fever.

This is a similar test to the above, using the toxin of the scarlet fever streptococcus in place of diphtheria toxin.

3. **Tuberculin tests.** The basis of the various tests for tuberculous infection is tuberculin. This is an extract obtained from tubercle bacilli and contains some of their toxins. The fact that it has been used in treatment in the past has already been mentioned.

The *Mantoux* test. This consists of the intradermal injection of 0·1 ml. of 1 in 10,000 dilution of Old Tuberculin into the forearm. In a positive reaction an area of redness and swelling develops at the site of inoculation within a few hours and reaches its maximum in twenty-four to forty-eight hours. If negative, subsequent tests may be carried out with stronger solutions. If negative, to 1 in 10,000 stronger solutions, e.g. 1 in 1000 to 1 in 100, may be employed.

This test is interpreted on a different basis to the tests for diphtheria and scarlet fever. Firstly, a distinction must be made between tuberculous infection and tuberculous disease. Sooner or later tubercle bacilli gain entrance to the body of almost every individual, but it is only in a few that active clinical tuberculous disease develops.

A positive reaction means that an individual has been infected by the tubercle bacillus at some time which may or may not have produced evidence of disease. By this infection he has been rendered sensitive or allergic to the toxins of the tubercle bacillus and the positive Mantoux test is an allergic reaction in the skin to the proteins contained in these toxins.

A positive reaction in young children often indicates active tuberculous disease. Except in special circumstances, a negative reaction indicates that there has been no tuberculous infection.

*Patch tests.* These are similar in principle and consist of the application to the surface of the skin of a patch of material saturated with tuberculin. This is left in position for 24 hours. Local redness and swelling indicate a positive reaction.

I

## Sera

The term serum used in therapeutics refers to the blood serum of an animal which has been rendered immune to a disease by means of a vaccine or toxin. Sometimes, also, serum is obtained from a human being who is convalescent from, or has previously had, a particular disease. Such sera, therefore, contain antibodies to the disease which have the power either of neutralizing the toxins or destroying the bacteria which cause the condition. They may be either:

1. Anti-toxic.

2. Anti-bacterial.

Because they contain antibodies "ready made" by another animal and the individual to whom they are given takes no part in the formation of these antibodies, they are described as producing "Passive Immunity".

Unfortunately it is not possible to produce sera which are effective against all organisms. Further, the introduction of chemotherapy and antibiotics have reduced considerably the use of certain sera, for example, anti-streptococcal serum and meningococcus antitoxin. A type of the former (scarlatina antitoxin) was used in the treatment of scarlet fever.

Among the more important sera are:

> Diphtheria antitoxin.
> Tetanus antitoxin.
> Gas gangrene antitoxin.
> Scarlatina antitoxin.
> Meningococcus antitoxin.
> Anti-anthrax serum (Sclavo's serum).
> Anti-dysentery serum.

Serum may be used (1) as a prophylactic agent after exposure to infection in order to prevent an attack or to minimize its severity, or (2) in the treatment of established disease.

Immunity acquired as a result of an infection lasts for a considerable period and often for a lifetime. Active immunity produced by a vaccine may last several years, but passive immunity obtained by the injection of a serum is of short duration which rarely exceeds a few weeks.

Sera may be administered by the subcutaneous, intramuscular, intravenous, intraperitoneal or intrathecal routes. The rate of absorption is most rapid when the intravenous route is used and this method is also of advantage when large doses have to be given. Intramuscular injection produces quicker results than subcutaneous.

*Serum sickness.* Because serum contains protein which is foreign in character to that of the individual receiving it, allergic reactions are sometimes observed 8 to 12 days after its administration. These consist of pyrexia, joint pains, rashes such as urticaria (wheals), erythema (general redness), etc. This condition is known as serum sickness and may be relieved by injections of adrenaline (1 in 1000), 5 to 15 minims (up to 1 ml.), and applications of calamine lotion if the rash is irritating. Antihistamine drugs are also given.

Modern methods of preparing serum have, however, reduced the amount of protein present to a minimum and reactions are not so common as formerly.

**Anaphylactic shock.** This is a severe type of allergic reaction. If a patient has at any time had an injection of horse serum, in any form, great care must be taken if another dose is given, as the individual is rendered over-sensitive to the proteins contained in horse serum. This over-sensitivity takes about ten days to develop and persists for a very long time. Once it has developed a second injection of serum may cause immediate and severe collapse or even sudden death. These symptoms are known as anaphylactic shock. Asthmatic patients are often sensitive to the injection of horse serum, and for these reasons, all patients should be asked if they suffer from asthma or if they have previously had serum, before the injection is given.

Adrenaline (1 in 1000), 5 to 15 minims (up to 1 ml.), is injected subcutaneously without delay. This may be followed by an intravenous antihistamine, e.g. diphenhydramine ('Benadryl') 10 mg., and if necessary intravenous hydrocortisone, 100 mg. in 500 ml. saline. If the symptoms do not abate the dose may be repeated. The foot of the bed should be raised, so that the head is low, and hot blankets and hot-water bottles applied.

Artificial respiration may be necessary.

Persons known to be sensitive are desensitized by giving a series of small amounts before the main dose, e.g. 0·5 ml., 1 ml., 2 ml., 5 ml. at intervals of 5 minutes.

In cases of diphtheria which have previously had antitoxin, a preliminary intramuscular injection of 1 ml. followed 6 hours later by the full intramuscular dose of serum has been found satisfactory. Adrenaline should always be at hand in case of emergency.

## Diphtheria antitoxin

This may be given subcutaneously, intramuscularly or intravenously. When large doses are used, the latter method is preferable. The dose is ordered in units according to the severity of the case, irrespective of the age of the patient, and may be repeated in 12 to 24 hours, e.g.:

| | |
|---|---|
| In mild cases and nasal diphtheria | 8000 units. |
| For moderately severe cases | 16,000 units. |
| For severe cases and laryngeal diphtheria | 24,000 to 100,000 units. |

## Scarlatina antitoxin

The dose is measured in millilitres, i.e. 10 to 30 ml.

It may be used in the treatment of scarlet fever.

**The Schultz-Charlton Reaction.** A small dose (0·2 ml.) of diluted scarlatina antitoxin is injected directly into the skin (intradermally) when the rash is present. If the rash is due to scarlet fever the skin around the site of injection becomes blanched and the rash disappears in that area.

## Tetanus antitoxin

Anti-tetanic serum may be used prophylactically and for the treatment of the disease.

*Prophylaxis.* The incidence of tetanus has been greatly reduced by giving appropriate doses of antitoxin without delay to all cases of accidental wounds, in particular those contaminated with road dirt. The minimum dose is 3000 units. In extensive and badly contaminated wounds it is repeated in a week.

A preliminary test dose for serum sensitivity of 0·2 ml. should be given first, followed by the remainder in 30 minutes if there is no reaction.

*Treatment.* Once the disease has developed, the only hope of success is to administer repeated large doses of antitoxin, e.g.

Initial dose:              25,000 to 100,000 units intravenously.

Repeated daily dose:  50,000 units

Total dosage:            300,000 to 400,000 units.

Sometimes, doses of 30,000 units are given intrathecally after the removal of an equivalent amount of cerebrospinal fluid. (The above doses refer to International units. U.S.A. units are twice the strength of the International unit.)

The symptoms of tetanus are caused by the toxins of the germ in the wound spreading up the nerves (or possibly by the blood-stream) to the brain and spinal cord. Once they have reached the central nervous system, the toxins become "fixed" in the tissues and are unaffected by antitoxin. The effect of the latter is to neutralize any more toxin manufactured in the wound and to render it harmless before it can reach the central nervous system.

At the same time, the spasms are controlled by sedatives such as pentothal, phenobarbitone, chlorpromazine, bromethol ('Avertin') or paraldehyde, the last two being given per rectum. Muscle relaxants 'Myanesin' may be given.

## The prevention of tetanus

In view of its high mortality the prevention of tetanus is of great importance and prophylactic measures are essential in most wounds due to trauma, especially in agricultural and garage workers. Individuals may be divided into two main groups:

1. *Immune*, i.e. those who have received three injections of tetanus vaccine within five years. A subsequent boosting dose will have given a further period of five years immunity.

Procedure: Such casualties only require a further 0·5 ml. of tetanus vaccine intramuscularly.

2. *Non-immune*, i.e. (*a*) those who have never received a full course of tetanus vaccine or who have not received a boosting dose within five years; (*b*) if more than a week has elapsed since a previous dose of tetanus antitoxin.

Procedure: (i) Provided non-immune patients have never had any type of serum before and have no history of allergic disease, they should be given not less than 1500 units of tetanus antitoxin at once.

(ii) If serum sensitivity is likely to be present, give test dose of 0·2 ml. antitoxin subcutaneously and wait 30 minutes before the remainder of the dose is given.

(iii) In allergic subjects the test dose of antitoxin should be diluted ten times with saline and 0·2 ml. of this mixture given. If no symptoms develop give 0·2 ml. undiluted toxin followed by the full dose in 30 minutes as in (ii). If allergic shock symptoms develop the patient should be kept warm, lying down and given 1 ml. of 1 in 1000 adrenaline intramuscularly. An anti-histamine may be required. If shock symptoms have developed wait until these have subsided (6 to 12 hours) then proceed as in (ii).

(iv) Following the administration of antitoxin the patient should be instructed to have a course of tetanus vaccine viz:

    0·5 ml. six weeks later.

    0·5 ml. six to twelve weeks later.

    0·5 ml. six to eighteen months later with subsequent boosting doses at intervals of five years.

It is important that the patient should have a record card indicating the treatment which has been given.

## Gas gangrene antitoxin

This may be given prophylactically to compound fractures or cases with dirt-contaminated wounds, at the same time as tetanus antitoxin. It is also used in the treatment of established gas gangrene. It is sometimes given in certain acute abdominal emergencies such as intestinal obstruction, especially when the bowel is gangrenous, and in peritonitis.

    Dose: (prophylactic)  4000 units.

           (therapeutic)  10,000 to 20,000 units by intravenous or intramuscular injection.

### Anti-anthrax serum (Sclavo's serum)

Repeated intravenous or intramuscular injections of 30 ml. are given. Good results are also obtained with neoarsphenamine, sulphonamides and penicillin which are usually more easily available than serum.

## Anti-dysentery serum

The dysentery bacilli may be divided into several types of which the most important are the Shiga group and the Flexner group. Anti-serum to both types is available either separately or mixed (polyvalent serum).

Doses up to 40 ml., or more, daily are given by intravenous or intramuscular injection.

Serum is of no value in the treatment of amœbic dysentery, for which emetine (page 80) is used.

## Anti-snake venom serum

This is used in the treatment of snake-bite and usually contains antibodies to cobra and viper venoms. The dose is 20-50 ml. intravenously.

## Convalescent serum and human Gamma Globulin

Human gamma globulin is used particularly in the prophylaxis of measles. It has also been employed in the prevention of poliomyelitis and rubella (1·5 gram to women who have been exposed to rubella during the first four months of pregnancy.)

## Measles prophylaxis

Serum collected from adult patients who are convalescent from the disease (convalescent serum) or who have suffered from measles in childhood (adult serum) contains antibodies to the virus. If this serum is administered to an individual who has been in contact with measles and who is incubating the disease, it has the power to prevent the development of the malady, or at least to modify its severity.

If the serum is given early in the incubation period, the disease is prevented (sero-prevention). If given after four days of the incubation period have elapsed, the disease is modified, and a mild attack occurs (sero-modification). The immunity conferred by sero-prevention only lasts for a few weeks and when it has passed off the individual is again liable to contract measles, if re-exposed to the infection. That following sero-modification of the disease is permanent.

In view of the prevalence of measles it is therefore preferable that a patient should acquire permanent immunity by suffering from a modified attack which is unlikely to prove serious, unless some other condition makes postponement essential. In very rare cases jaundice may follow the injection of convalescent serum after an interval of a number of weeks.

**Gamma globulin.** Although the above account illustrates the principles employed in the prophylaxis of measles actual serum is now rarely used. Instead, that portion of the serum which contains the necessary antibodies known as gamma globulin is given. This is prepared from a pool of serum obtained from not less than a thousand individuals who have not necessarily suffered from a recent infection.

This is therapeutically active because the serum of most adults contain antibodies.

The dose is up to 1·5 gram.

A special anti-hæmophilic globulin (AHG) is available for use in hæmophilia.

### Protein shock therapy

Protein shock therapy or non-specific protein therapy is a form of treatment which is sometimes encountered.

It is likely to be most useful in diseases of an allergic nature and appears to act in some way which enables the patient to desensitize himself to the substance causing the allergic state. How this actually happens is not clear, but the results produced are due to the protein contained in the preparation used.

Numerous substances have been employed for this purpose and are generally given by intravenous or intramuscular injection, which may be followed by a transient febrile reaction, e.g.

Peptone.
Sterile proteins.
T.A.B. vaccine (intravenously).

Similar results are also produced by giving the patient an intramuscular injection of his own blood immediately after its withdrawal from a vein (auto-hæmo-therapy).

# CHAPTER 19

# RADIOACTIVE ISOTOPES

Although not many doctors and nurses will handle these substances personally their increasing use in medicine justifies a brief reference to the subject which, however, cannot be fully understood without extensive knowledge of atomic physics. Nevertheless some of the more simple aspects can be generally appreciated.

1. Basically, matter consists of a number of individual elements alone or in combination.

2. Elements consist of atoms.

3. An atom consists of a central nucleus with a number of electrons revolving round it.

4. The nucleus of an atom consists of two types of particles, (*a*) protons, (*b*) neutrons.

5. The number of protons in the nucleus of an atom equals the number of electrons which revolve round it.

6. The chemical properties and characteristics of each element are determined by the number of electrons in its atom.

7. Under certain circumstances the number of neutrons in the atom of an element may be varied. Although the element will then have the same general chemical characteristics its atom will be unstable and it will emit radiation of particles and rays, i.e. it becomes a radioactive isotope of the element.

8. Certain elements occur in a natural state as a mixture of normal atoms and their radioactive isotopes, e.g. uranium and radium. Radioactive isotopes of other elements can be produced by subjecting the normal atom of that element to the action of an 'atom-smashing machine'.

9. In some instances the isotopes are very unstable and have a short life, that is, after emitting their radiation at a rapid rate the atoms soon return to normal. In others, this process may take days, weeks or many years before the radioactivity ceases, although in fact it is diminishing at a steady rate all the time. This loss of activity is described in terms of 'half-life'.

For example radioactive iodine has a 'half-life' of 8 days which means that at the end of each eight day period only half of the radio-activity present at the commencement of that period remains.

10. Radioactivity can be detected and measured by special apparatus, (a) Geiger counter, (b) scintillation counter.

11. Living cells cannot distinguish between the normal element and the radioactive isotope. If, therefore, a tissue takes up the isotope its presence can be detected and measured by a 'counter'.

These facts are applied to medicine in the following ways,

1. Research and diagnosis.  2. Therapy.

A great deal of information has been obtained by isotope research on the metabolism and distribution of various substances throughout the body, e.g. the absorption of iodine, its concentration in the thyroid gland and use in the formation of thyroxine. Subsequently, the release and distribution of radioactive thyroxine into the bloodstream has been demonstrated.

Although deep X-rays and radium remain the most useful and generally employed methods of radiation therapy for appropriate conditions, radioactive isotopes may be used in certain circumstances, e.g. malignant tumours of the tongue and bladder which were formerly treated by implanting radium needles may now be dealt with by using smaller needles or wires containing isotopes which are more easily handled. Liquid solutions can also be used, e.g. radioactive gold (Gold[198]) solution may be introduced into the pleural cavity in certain cases of malignant pleural effusion.

Other radioactive isotopes in use are:

(a) Iodine[131], which given orally in appropriate dosage is an effective method of treating some cases of thyrotoxicosis.

The uptake of a small dose of radioactive iodine by the thyroid gland is a valuable test for thyrotoxicosis.

(*b*) Phosphorus[32] is used in the treatment of polycythæmia vera, a condition in which there is an excess of red blood corpuscles. This substance acts by depressing the overactive bone marrow.

## The use of isotopes in hospital.

All forms of radioactivity, except in the most carefully controlled and minute doses may affect health adversely. An individual who has been given a radioactive isotope will continue to excrete this in the urine and fæces for some time. The radiation from these excreta might be dangerous to others who come in contact with them. Special precautions are, therefore, necessary. A specially screened storage room is essential. All urine, etc. must be collected and stored for several days or even weeks until the radioactivity has decayed sufficiently for it to be disposed of in the normal sewage system. Similar precautions are necessary for any contaminated bedding or clothing.

A hospital unit handling these substances will have special rules and provided they are strictly followed by the staff and patients, the administration of these substances is quite simple and will probably play an increasingly important part in the therapy of the future.

# CHAPTER 20

# WEIGHTS, MEASURES, PRESCRIPTIONS AND MISCELLANEOUS TABLES

The English systems of weights and measures are complicated. In addition to the Imperial or avoirdupois measures used in everyday life, there is a system of Apothecaries' weights employed exclusively in dispensing.

Full tables of weights and measures will be found on page 261 but in practice the approximate equivalents are used rather than the exact scientific figures indicated on page 274.

## THE METRIC SYSTEM

The Metric System is used on the Continent and is also being employed increasingly in the United States. It is frequently encountered in this country and almost every new drug is ordered by weight in grams or milligrams, and by fluid measure in millilitres (cubic centimetres and millilitres may be regarded as identical in volume). The nurse must, therefore, be familiar with these measures and must be able to convert doses ordered in Apothecaries' Measure into the Metric System, and vice versa.

### Metric weights

$$\begin{aligned}
\text{10 milligrams (mg.)} &= \text{1 centigram} = 0 \cdot 01 \ (\tfrac{1}{100}) \text{ gram} \\
\left.\begin{array}{l}\text{1000 milligrams} \\ \text{100 centigrams}\end{array}\right\} &= \text{1 gram (G.)} \\
\text{1000 grams} &= \text{1 kilogram}
\end{aligned}$$

### Metric volume

$$\begin{aligned}
\left.\begin{array}{l}\text{1 millilitre (mil or ml)} \\ \text{1 cubic centimetre (c.c.)}\end{array}\right\} &= 0 \cdot 001 \text{ litre} \\
\text{1000 millilitres} &= \text{1 litre}
\end{aligned}$$

### Metric length

The standard measure of length is the metre (about 39 inches).

1 centimetre $= \tfrac{1}{100}$ part of a metre (0·01 metre).

1 millimetre $= \tfrac{1}{10}$ part of a centimetre (0·001 metre).

## Equivalents

The following are some of the important approximate equivalents between the Imperial and Apothecaries' Systems and the Metric System. (see also page 276)

| | | |
|---|---|---|
| **Weight** | ¼ grain | = 15 milligrams (0·015 gram) |
| | 1 grain | = 60 milligrams (0·06 gram) |
| | 1½ grains | = 100 milligrams (0·1 gram) |
| | 15 grains | = 1 gram (1·0 gram) |
| | 1 ounce | = 30 grams |
| | 1 pound | = 450 grams |
| | 2·2 pounds | = 1 kilogram |
| **Volume** | 15 minims | = 1 mil (c.c.) |
| | 1 fluid drachm | = 4 ml. |
| | 1 fluid ounce | = 30 ml. |
| | 1 pint | = 570 ml. |
| | 1¾ pints | = 1 litre |

## Conversion of Metric and Imperial Weights, etc.

The most important approximate figures are: To convert:

### Weight

| | |
|---|---|
| grains to grams | × 0·065 |
| grams to grains | × 15 |
| grams to ounces | × 0·03 |
| kilograms to pounds | × 2·2 |

### Fluid

| | |
|---|---|
| millilitres (c.c.) to minims | × 15 |
| minims to millilitres | × 0·06 |
| pints to litres | × 0·57 |

## SOLUTIONS

The nurse is sometimes called upon to make up solutions of a certain strength from other stronger solutions or solid drugs. This practice involves various mathematical calculations in which accuracy is obviously of great importance.

Solutions may be:

1. Hypertonic, Isotonic, Hypotonic (see page 107).
2. Expressed as a percentage.
3. Expressed (*a*) as grains to an ounce.
        (*b*) as minims or drachms to a pint.
        (*c*) in the Metric System.
4. Saturated solutions.

## Saturated solutions

A saturated solution is one which contains as much solid as it is capable of dissolving; any additional amount of solid remains undissolved as a sediment.

It will be clear from experience that some substances (e.g. sodium chloride, common salt) are very soluble and will dissolve in a small amount of water. Others are less soluble, dissolve slowly and require a much greater quantity of water; while some are insoluble.

Further, the rate and degree of solubility is usually increased when the temperature of the water is raised.

## Percentage solutions

A percentage solution expresses the number of parts of a drug in one hundred parts of the final solution. The abbreviations "per cent" or "%" are used to denote this. For example:

A 5 per cent solution of dextrose contains:

| 5 parts | of dextrose in | 100 parts | of the solution |
|---|---|---|---|
| 1 part | ,, ,, ,, | 20 ,, | ,, ,, ,, |
| 5 grams | ,, ,, ,, | 100 ml. | ,, ,, ,, |

*Example.* (i) *To find the amount of dextrose required to make a pint (20 fluid ounces) of 5 per cent solution.*

100 fl. oz. of 5% solution will contain 5 oz.    dextrose

| 1 | ,, ,, ,, | ,, | ,, | ,, | $\frac{5}{100}$ oz. | ,, |
|---|---|---|---|---|---|---|
| 20 | ,, ,, ,, | ,, | ,, | ,, | $\frac{5}{100} \times 20$ oz. | ,, |
| 20 | ,, ,, ,, | ,, | ,, | ,, | 1 oz. | ,, |

(ii) *To find the amount of sodium chloride required to make a pint of 0·9 per cent solution (normal saline).*

100 fl. oz. of 0·9% solution will contain 0·9 oz. sodium chloride

| 1 | ,, ,, ,, | ,, | ,, | ,, | $\frac{0·9 \text{ oz.}}{100}$ ,, ,, |
|---|---|---|---|---|---|---|
| 20 | ,, ,, ,, | ,, | ,, | ,, | $\frac{0·9}{100} \times 20$ oz. ,, |
| 20 | ,, ,, ,, | ,, | ,, | ,, | $\frac{0·9 \times 20 \times 437·5 \text{ grains}}{100}$ sodium chloride |

(because 1 oz. avoir. contains 437·5 grains)

20 fl. oz. of 0·9% solution will contain 78·75 grains sodium chloride

N.B.—1 pint of 1 per cent solution contains 87·5 grains of any solid, therefore:

1 pint of 0·9 per cent $\left(\frac{9}{10}\%\right)$ solution contains $87·5 \times \frac{9}{10} = 78·75$ grains.

(This is another method of obtaining the same result. In practice, the approximate figure of 80 grains in one pint is accepted as a round number to make up normal saline.)

When dealing with small amounts of fluid and using minims as the measure of volume, it must be remembered that:

480 minims of water weigh 437·5 grains (1 oz. avoir.)

Therefore:

since a 1% solution contains 1 part of solid in 100 parts of solution

1 „ „ 1 grain „ „ „ 100 grains of solution

and 100 grains of water measure $\dfrac{480}{437·5} = 110$ minims

1% solution contains 1 grain of solid in 110 minims of solution.

*Example. To find the amount of atropine sulphate required to make 440 minims of ½ per cent atropine sulphate drops.* (This amount is just less than 1 fluid ounce, or 480 minims, and is frequently supplied for convenience in calculation.)

110 minims of solution contain ½ grain atropine sulphate

440 „ „ „ „ $\dfrac{1}{2} \times \dfrac{440}{110}$ grains „ „

440 „ „ „ „ 2 grains „ „

Percentage calculations in the Metric System are simple. For example: a 1% solution is prepared by dissolving 1 gram of a solid in water and making the amount up to 100 ml.

i.e. 100 ml. of solution contains 1 gram = 1 per cent

100 ml. „ „ „ 2·5 gram = 2·5 per cent

## To make solutions from tablets of known strength

For convenience a number of drugs commonly used in making solutions are often supplied in tablets (solvellæ) of definite strengths, e.g.

Sodium chloride . . 40 or 80 grain tablets

Mercury biniodide ⎱
Mercury perchloride ⎰ . 8·75 grain tablets

*Example.* (*i*) *To make* 1 *pint of saline containing* 80 *grains per pint.*

1 tablet of 80 grains or 2 tablets of 40 grains each are dissolved in water and the solution made up to 1 pint.

(*ii*) *To make* ½ *pint of* 20 *per cent* (*hypertonic*) *saline.*

It will be recalled that a 1% solution contains 87·5 grains in 1 pint. Therefore:

1 pint of 20% solution contains 87·5 ×20=1750 grains

½ ,, ,, ,, ,, ,, $\dfrac{1750}{2}$ = 875 grains

Number of 40-grain tablets required $=\dfrac{875}{40}=$ 22 approx.

(*iii*) *To make* 1 *pint of* 1 *in* 1000 *solution of mercury biniodide, using tablets containing* 8·75 *grains.*

1 in 1000 solution =a 0·1 per cent solution

1% solution =87·5 grains in 1 pint of solution

0·1% ,, =8·75 grains ,, 1 pint ,, ,,

Therefore:

1 tablet of 8·75 grains in 1 pint makes 1 in 1000 solution.

*N.B.*—The addition of 3 parts of water to 1 part of a 1 in 1000 solution will make a 1 in 4000 solution.

## Dosage of hypodermic tablets

Sometimes solutions of drugs given by hypodermic injection are prepared from tablets of appropriate strength, e.g.:

Morphine sulphate is usually supplied in tablets of—

$\frac{1}{12}$, $\frac{1}{8}$, $\frac{1}{6}$, $\frac{1}{4}$, $\frac{1}{3}$ and ½ grain.

Atropine sulphate is supplied in tablets of—

$\frac{1}{200}$, $\frac{1}{150}$, $\frac{1}{100}$ and $\frac{1}{75}$ grain.

Not infrequently, however, supplies of tablets of the exact dose ordered may not be available and it is necessary to obtain the dose from tablets of a different strength. In view of the fact that most of the drugs given by hypodermic injection are very powerful, the strictest accuracy must be observed in making calculations.

*Example.* (i) *To prepare an injection of morphine sulphate $\frac{1}{6}$ grain from a supply of tablets containing $\frac{1}{4}$ grain each.*

Dissolve $\frac{1}{4}$-grain tablet in 12 minims of sterile water.

12 minims of solution contains $\frac{1}{4}$ grain

     1 minim   ,,   ,,   ,,   $\frac{1}{4} \times \frac{1}{12} = \frac{1}{48}$ grain

Since    $\frac{1}{48}$ grain is contained in   1 minim

     1   ,,   ,,   ,,   ,, 48 minims

Therefore $\frac{1}{6}$  ,,   ,,   ,,   ,, $\frac{48}{6} = 8$ minims

The amount 12 minims in which to dissolve the tablet is selected because it is the smallest convenient figure which is exactly divisible by 4 and 6.

If, for example, it was necessary to obtain a dose of $\frac{1}{5}$ grain from tablets containing $\frac{1}{3}$ grain of a given drug, the amount of water used as a solvent would be 15 minims, because 15 is the smallest convenient amount exactly divisible by 5 and 3.

The aim should be to produce an injection of 5 to 15 minims, smaller amounts being difficult to measure accurately and larger ones being inconvenient to administer.

(ii) *To prepare an injection containing $\frac{1}{100}$ grain of atropine sulphate from a supply of tablets each containing $\frac{1}{150}$ grain.*

In this instance the problem is to produce a solution containing a greater dosage than a single dose of the tablet supplied.

As $\frac{1}{150}$ grain is less than $\frac{1}{100}$ grain it is necessary to use two tablets ($\frac{1}{150} \times 2 = \frac{1}{75}$ grain).

Therefore: dissolve two tablets of $\frac{1}{150}$ grain in 10 minims of sterile water.

    10 minims of solution contain $\frac{1}{150} \times 2 = \frac{1}{75}$ grain

     1 minim ,,   ,,   ,, $\frac{1}{75} \times \frac{1}{10} = \frac{1}{750}$ grain

   $\frac{1}{750}$ grain is contained in   1 minim

     1   ,,   ,,   ,,   ,, 750 minims

   $\frac{1}{100}$  ,,   ,,   ,,   ,, $\frac{750}{100} = 7.5$ minims

Therefore: dissolve two tablets of $\frac{1}{150}$ grain in 10 minims of sterile water and inject 7.5 ($7\frac{1}{2}$) minims.

(iii) *To prepare an injection of $\frac{1}{75}$ grain atropine sulphate from a supply of tablets containing $\frac{1}{100}$ grain.*

As in the previous example, dissolve two tablets of $\frac{1}{100}$ grain in 12 minims.

$$12 \text{ minims contain } 2 \times \tfrac{1}{100} = \tfrac{1}{50} \text{ grain}$$
$$1 \text{ minim contains } \tfrac{1}{50} \times \tfrac{1}{12} = \tfrac{1}{600} \text{ grain}$$

If   1 grain is contained in 600 minims

then:  $\frac{1}{75}$ ,, ,, ,, ,, $\frac{600}{75} = 8$ minims

Therefore: to obtain $\frac{1}{75}$ grain from a tablet containing $\frac{1}{100}$ grain, dissolve two $\frac{1}{100}$ grain tablets in 12 minims and inject 8 minims of the solution.

There is an alternative method of making the above calculations which some may find easier.

(i) *To obtain a dose of $\frac{1}{6}$ grain from tablets containing $\frac{1}{4}$ grain.*

$\frac{1}{4}$ grain is contained in 1 tablet

1 ,, ,, ,, ,, 4 tablets

$\frac{1}{6}$ ,, ,, ,, ,, $\frac{4}{6} = \frac{2}{3}$ tablets

Therefore: if 1 tablet is dissolved in 12 minims

$\frac{2}{3}$ tablet is contained in $12 \times \frac{2}{3} = 8$ minims of solution

(ii) *To obtain a dose of $\frac{1}{100}$ grain from tablets of $\frac{1}{150}$ grain.*

$\frac{1}{150}$ grain is contained in 1 tablet

1 ,, ,, ,, ,, 150 tablets

$\frac{1}{100}$ ,, ,, ,, ,, $\frac{150}{100} = 1 \cdot 5$ ($1\frac{1}{2}$) tablets

Therefore: if 2 tablets are dissolved in 10 minims

1·5 tablets are contained in $\frac{10}{2} \times 1 \cdot 5 = 7\frac{1}{2}$ minim solution

(iii) *To obtain a dose of $\frac{1}{75}$ grain from tablets containing $\frac{1}{100}$ grain.*

$\frac{1}{100}$ grain is contained in 1 tablet

1 ,, ,, ,, ,, 100 tablets

$\frac{1}{75}$ ,, ,, ,, ,, $\frac{100}{75} = \frac{4}{3}$ tablets

Therefore: if 2 tablets are dissolved in 12 minims

$\frac{4}{3}$ tablets are contained in $\frac{12}{2} \times \frac{4}{3} = 8$ minims of solution

## To obtain an exact dosage from a percentage solution

*Example. To obtain $\frac{1}{4}$ grain of morphine sulphate from a $2 \cdot 5\%$ solution.*
By definition (page 244):

1% solution contains 1 grain in 110 minims

$2 \cdot 5\%$ ,, ,, ,, $2 \cdot 5$ ,, ,, 110 minims

i.e. 1 grain is contained in $\dfrac{110}{2 \cdot 5}$ minims

$\frac{1}{4}$ ,, ,, ,, ,, $\dfrac{110 \times \frac{1}{4}}{2 \cdot 5} = 11$ minims

## Dilution of lotions and other solutions

The strengths of various solutions may be expressed either as a percentage or as 1 part of the substance in a definite volume of the solution, e.g.

$$
\begin{aligned}
1 \text{ in} \quad 5 \text{ solution} &= 20 \text{ per cent} \\
1 \text{ in} \quad 10 \quad ,, \quad &= 10 \text{ per cent} \\
1 \text{ in} \quad 40 \quad ,, \quad &= 2\cdot5 \text{ per cent } (2\tfrac{1}{2} \text{ per cent}) \\
1 \text{ in} \quad 80 \quad ,, \quad &= 1\cdot25 \text{ per cent} \\
1 \text{ in} \quad 100 \quad ,, \quad &= 1 \text{ per cent} \\
1 \text{ in} \quad 500 \quad ,, \quad &= 0\cdot2 \text{ per cent} \\
1 \text{ in} \quad 1000 \quad ,, \quad &= 0\cdot1 \text{ per cent}
\end{aligned}
$$

*Example.* (*i*) *To make 1 pint of 1 in 80 solution from a 1 in 40 stock solution.*

Take ½ pint of 1 in 40 stock solution and add water to make up 1 pint.

(*ii*) *To make 10 fluid ounces of a 1 per cent solution from a 1 in 40 stock solution.*

Since 1 part of drug is contained in 40 parts of stock solution and we require 1 part of the drug in 100 parts of solution (1%), take 40 parts of stock and make up to 100 parts with water.

Then: 100 parts of new solution will contain 40 parts of stock solution

1 part of new solution will contain $\frac{40}{100}$ parts of stock solution

10 fluid ounces of new solution will contain $\frac{40}{100} \times 10 =$ 4 fluid ounces of stock solution

Therefore: take 4 fluid ounces of 1 in 40 stock solution and dilute to 10 fluid ounces of water to make a 1 per cent solution.

## THE PRESCRIPTION

A prescription is a formula stating the ingredients of a remedy with directions for its preparation and administration. (The term is derived from the Latin, *præ* = before; *scribo* = I write.)

The prescriptions of the present time tend to be much simpler than formerly and, in hospital in particular, considerable use is made of standard mixtures. This saves much time and labour in a pharmacy. However, the nurse will meet full prescriptions from time to time and should understand their meaning and construction.

Every drug or application ordered is, strictly speaking, a prescription, and in many instances is written in Latin, in the form of standard abbreviations. The directions for the administration may be either in English or in Latin.

The classical prescription consists of a number of parts:

The name of the patient.
The superscription.
The inscription.
The subscription.
The signature.
The name of the prescriber and the date of the prescription.

These terms can best be explained by examining a typical prescription.

William Smith, Esq.

> ℞. Potassii chloratis . . . . gr. x
> Liquoris ferri perchloridi . . m. xv
> Glycerini . . . . . m. xxx
> Aquam . . . . . . ad ℥ i
>        Fiat mistura.        Mitte ℥x.
>        Signetur ℥ i, ter die sumenda, post cibos.

29th February, 1900                    John Jones, M.D.

Using abbreviations this would also be correctly written as:

William Smith, Esq.

> ℞. Pot. chlor. . . . . . gr. x
> Liq. ferri perchlor. . . . m. xv
> Glycer. . . . . . m. xxx
> Aq. . . . . . . . ad ℥ i
>        F.M.        M. ℥x
>        Sign. ℥ i, t.d.s., p.c.

29/2/00                    John Jones, M.D.

The complete English translation of the above prescription would therefore be:

William Smith, Esq.
   Take thou (a direction to the Pharmacist)
     of potassium chlorate    .   .   .   .   10 grains
     of solution of iron perchloride   .  .  15 minims
     of glycerin .   .   .   .   .   .   30 minims
     Put (or add) water up to one ounce
     Let a mixture be made.       Send 10 ounces.
Let it be labelled one ounce (two tablespoonfuls) to be taken three
   times a day, after meals.
   29th February, 1900.          John Jones, M.D.

The above prescription can be analysed in the following way.

**Name of patient.** This is obvious. The address may also be included. It is also permissible to put the patient's name at the end of the prescription.

**Superscription.** This is a sort of heading in the form of an instruction to the pharmacist. The symbol R is used and is an abbreviation of the Latin, *recipe* = take (thou).

**The inscription.** This is the prescription proper and is a list of the various ingredients, together with the amount of each. When written in Latin, it is expressed grammatically in the genitive case because it qualifies the amount 10 grains, i.e. 10 grains of potassium chlorate.

**The subscription.** This is an instruction to the pharmacist. It states the form which the preparation is to take and the amount to be dispensed.

Fiat mistura (F.M.) means "Let a mixture be made."
Mitte ℥x means "Send 10 ounces."
Fiat pilula would mean "Let a pill be made."
Fiat lotio would mean "Let a lotion be made."

**The signature.** This does not mean the signature of the prescriber but refers to the directions to be given to the patient. Signetur or Sign. means "Let it be labelled" and the subsequent instructions may be written in Latin, in abbreviated form or in English.

The prescription is completed by the addition of the doctor's name or initials and the date. When drugs controlled by the Dangerous Drugs Act are included, the total amount of the drugs to be supplied must be stated.

In view of the fact that the signs ʒ (drachm) and ℥ (ounce) are apt to be misread the modern tendency is to prescribe solids in grains (gr.) and ounces (oz.), and fluids in minims (m) and fluid ounces (fl. oz.). Also ordinary numbers replace the roman numerals. When using the Metric System a gram is written as a capital G, and the millilitre (ml.) is often used instead of the cubic centimetre (c.c.) as a unit of volume.

## Latin phrases and abbreviations commonly used in prescribing

| | | |
|---|---|---|
| Ana | a̅a̅. | of each |
| Ante cibum (cibos) | a.c. | before food (meals) |
| Ad libitum | ad lib. | to the amount desired |
| Æquales | æq. | equal |
| Alternis diebus | alt. die. | alternate days (every other day) |
| Alternis noctibus | alt. noct. | alternate nights |
| Aqua | aq. | water |
| Bis die | b.d. | |
| Bis in die | b.i.d. | twice a day |
| Cras mane | c.m. | to-morrow morning |
| Cras nocte | c.n. | to-morrow night |
| Cum | c̄. | with |
| Ex aqua | ex. aq. | in water |
| Hac nocte | h.n. | this night |
| Mitte | m. | send |
| Nocte et mane | n. et m. (nmque) | night and morning |
| Omni mane | o.m. | every morning |
| Omni nocte | o.n. | every night |
| Parti affectæ | p.a. | to the affected part |
| Post cibum (cibos) | p.c. | after food (meals) |
| Pro oculis | p.oc. | for the eyes |
| Pro re nata | p.r.n. | as the occasion arises (to be repeated when required) |
| Quater in die | q.i.d. | four times a day |
| Quantum sufficiat | q.s. | a sufficient quantity |
| Repetatur | rep. | let it be repeated |
| Semissis | ss. or ſs. | half |
| Si opus sit | s.o.s. | if necessary (a single dose) |
| Statim | stat. | at once |
| Ter die sumendum | t.d.s. | to be taken three times a day |
| Ter in die | t.i.d. | three times a day |

## LATIN TERMINOLOGY

The fact that Latin is used, not only in connection with the official terminology of drugs but also in Anatomy and other branches of Medical Science, often adds to the difficulties of the student who has no knowledge of the language or its pronunciation. The following notes on the pronunciation usually employed and the grammar involved may be useful.

### Pronunciation

Among the main rules for the pronunciation of technical Latin and of English words derived from Latin are:

æ is pronounced "ee" as in æquales (equal)
                         spirochæte
                         mammæ (breasts)

œ is pronounced "ee" as in œdema (a very common mistake
                         is to call this "odema"!)
                         œsophagus
                         œstrin

-i (at the end of a word) is pronounced "i, long as in like"
                         e.g. ferri (of iron)

-ii (at the end of a word), first "i" short as in tin,
                         second "i" long as in like.
                         as in calcii (of calcium)
                              sodii (of sodium)

c is soft (i.e. like "s") before "e" and "i",
                         as in cerebrum
                         cinchophenum

c is hard (i.e. like "k") before "a", "o" and "u",
                         as in calomel
                         codeina
                         cuprum (copper)
                         cum (with)

g is soft (i.e. like "j") before "e" and "i",
                         as in Progestin
                         genital
                         gingivitis

g is hard (as in "go") before "a", "o" and "u",

as in gastric

goitre

gumma

## Grammar

The types of word commonly encountered are:

***Nouns :*** names of persons, places or things. In the nominative case (see below) many Latin nouns have the following endings:

| | | |
|---|---|---|
| -a | e.g. | aqua |
| -us | | spiritus |
| -um | | acidum |
| -as | | benzoas |
| -is | | cannabis |

***Adjectives :*** words which express qualities of nouns:

aqua calida  = hot water

aqua destillata  = distilled water

Frequently the Latin adjective has the same ending as the noun as in the examples above, but this is not always so, e.g. injectio hypodermica.

***Verbs :*** words which express an action or state. In the prescription the following are all verbs:

fiat (mistura) = let (a mixture) be made

mitte             = send

recipe           = take (thou)

***Prepositions :*** words denoting the relation of nouns to other words in the sentence:

per urethram = through or by the urethra

***Conjunctions :*** words connecting nouns or phrases:

et   = and (e.g. *Ferri et ammonii citras*—iron and ammonium citrate)

cum = with (e.g. *Hydrargyrum cum creta*, Mercury with chalk)

Nouns undergo certain changes in form: Thus there is usually a different ending to denote singular (one person or thing) and plural (more than one).

| | |
|---|---|
| aqua, water | aquæ, waters |
| acidum, acid | acida, acids |
| pessus, a pessary | pessi, pessaries |
| vapor, an inhalation | vapores, inhalations |

There is, however, no simple rule which can be given to indicate all the various changes which may occur.

The endings of nouns also change according to the case. The case of a noun depends on its relation to other words in the phrase or sentence, but the only two of importance in the present connection are the nominative and genitive cases. The former is the subject of the sentence, the latter answers the question "of what or whom". For example, in the description of a drug:

sodii sulphas = sulphate (nominative) of sodium (genitive).

It will be recalled that a prescription commences with the symbol ℞ (*recipe*—take thou), the rest of the prescription is therefore written in the genitive case, i.e.

| ℞ | sodii sulphatis |
|---|---|
| take thou | of sulphate of sodium (both words being in the genitive case, the genitive of sulphas being sulphatis) |

### THERMOMETRIC EQUIVALENTS
*Within Clinical Limits*

| ° C. | ° F. | ° C. | ° F. |
|---|---|---|---|
| 35·0 | 95·0 | 39·0 | 102·20 |
| 36·0 | 96·80 | 39·2 | 102·56 |
| 36·2 | 97·16 | 39·4 | 102·92 |
| 36·4 | 97·52 | 39·6 | 103·28 |
| 36·6 | 97·88 | 39·8 | 103·64 |
| 36·8 | 98·24 | 40·0 | 104·0 |
| 37·0 | 98·60 | 40·2 | 104·36 |
| 37·2 | 98·96 | 40·4 | 104·72 |
| 37·4 | 99·32 | 40·6 | 105·08 |
| 37·6 | 99·68 | 40·8 | 105·44 |
| 37·8 | 100·04 | 41·0 | 105·80 |
| 38·0 | 100·40 | 42·0 | 107·60 |
| 38·2 | 100·76 | 43·0 | 109·40 |
| 38·4 | 101·12 | 44·0 | 111·20 |
| 38·6 | 101·48 | | |
| 38·8 | 101·84 | | |

To convert °C. to °F. multiply by $\frac{9}{5}$ and add 32.
E.g. 37°C. $\times \frac{9}{5} = 66 \cdot 6 + 32 = 98 \cdot 6$°F.
To convert °F. to °C. subtract 32 and multiply by $\frac{5}{9}$.
E.g. 100°F.—32 = 68 $\times \frac{5}{9} = 37 \cdot 7$°C.

## WEIGHTS AND MEASURES

### AVOIRDUPOIS WEIGHT

| | | |
|---|---|---|
| 437·5 grains | = 1 ounce (oz.) | |
| 16 ounces | = 1 pound (lb.) | = 7000 grains |
| 14 pounds | = 1 stone (st.) | |
| 28 pounds | = 1 quarter (qr.) | |
| 4 quarters | = 1 hundredweight (cwt.) | = 112 lb. |
| 20 cwt. | = 1 ton | = 2,240 lb. |

### APOTHECARIES WEIGHT

| | | |
|---|---|---|
| 20 grains | = 1 scruple (Ɵ) | |
| 3 scruples | = 1 drachm (ʒi) | = 60 grains |
| 8 drachms | = 1 ounce (ʒi) | = 480 grains |

### APOTHECARIES FLUID MEASURES

| | | | |
|---|---|---|---|
| 60 minims | = 1 fluid drachm | | |
| 8 fluid drachms | = 1 fluid ounce | = 480 minims | |
| 20 fluid ounces | = 1 pint | = 160 drachms | = 9,600 minims |
| 2 pints | = 1 quart | | |
| 4 quarts | = 1 gallon | = 160 ounces | = 1,280 drachms |

N.B.—The term "scruple" is never used and the drachm is no longer "official" in the B.P.

### METRIC WEIGHTS

| | | |
|---|---|---|
| 10 milligrams | = 1 centigram | = 0·154 grains |
| 10 centigrams | = 1 decigram | = 1·543 ,, |
| 10 decigrams | = 1 gram | = 15·432 ,, |
| 10 grams | = 1 decagram | = 0·3527 oz. av. |
| 10 decagrams | = 1 hectogram | = 3·5274 ,, |
| 10 hectograms | = 1 kilogram (kilo) | = 2·2046 lb. |

### METRIC VOLUME OR CAPACITY

| | | |
|---|---|---|
| 10 centimils | = 1 decimil | = 1·6894 minims |
| 10 decimils | = 1 mil (c.c.) | = 16·8941 minims |
| 10 mils (c.c.) | = 1 centilitre | = 2·8157 fl. drachms |
| 100 mils (c.c.) | = 1 decilitre | = 3·5196 fl. oz. |
| 1000 mils (c.c.) | = 1 litre | = 1·7598 pints |

## Approximate Equivalents

### WEIGHTS—IMPERIAL TO METRIC

| Gr. | Gram | Gr. | Gram | Gr. | Gram |
|---|---|---|---|---|---|
| $\frac{1}{1000}$ | = 0·000065 | $\frac{1}{5}$ | = 0·013 | 15 | = 1·0 |
| $\frac{1}{200}$ | = 0·00032 | $\frac{1}{4}$ | = 0·016 | 20 | = 1·29 |
| $\frac{1}{120}$ | = 0·005 (0·5 mg.) | $\frac{1}{3}$ | = 0·02 (20 mg.) | 30 | = 2·0 |
| $\frac{1}{100}$ | = 0·00065 | $\frac{1}{2}$ | = 0·03 | 45 | = 3·0 |
| $\frac{1}{64}$ | = 0·001 (1 mg.) | $\frac{3}{4}$ | = 0·05 (50 mg.) | 60 | = 3·9 |
| $\frac{1}{50}$ | = 0·0013 | 1 | = 0·065 | 90 | = 6·0 |
| $\frac{1}{40}$ | = 0·0015 | $1\frac{1}{2}$ | = 0·1 (100 mg.) | 120 | = 7·8 |
| $\frac{1}{32}$ | = 0·002 (2 mg.) | 2 | = 0·12 | 150 | = 10·0 |
| $\frac{1}{25}$ | = 0·0025 | 3 | = 0·2 (200 mg.) | 180 | = 12·0 |
| $\frac{1}{20}$ | = 0·003 | 4 | = 0·25 | | |
| $\frac{1}{16}$ | = 0·004 (5 mg.) | 5 | = 0·3 | $\frac{1}{2}$ ounce (av.) | = 15·0 |
| $\frac{1}{12}$ | = 0·005 | 6 | = 0·4 | 1 ounce (av.) | = 30·0 |
| $\frac{1}{10}$ | = 0·0065 | 8 | = 0·5 | (or nearer 28·35) | |
| $\frac{1}{8}$ | = 0·008 | 10 | = 0·65 | 1 pound | = 453·59 |
| $\frac{1}{6}$ | = 0·01 (10 mg.) | 12 | = 0·8 | | |

### MEASURES—IMPERIAL TO METRIC

| Minims | ml. | Minims | ml. | Fluid oz. | ml. |
|---|---|---|---|---|---|
| $\frac{1}{2}$ | = 0·03 | 15 | = 0·9 or 1·0 | 1 | = 30·0 |
| 1 | = 0·06 | 20 | = 1·2 | 2 | = 60·0 |
| 2 | = 0·12 | 25 | = 1·5 | 4 | = 115·0 |
| 3 | = 0·2 | 30 | = 2·0 | 5 | = 140·0 |
| 4 | = 0·25 | 40 | = 2·5 | 6 | = 170·0 |
| 5 | = 0·3 | 45 | = 3·0 | 8 | = 230·0 |
| 6 | = 0·35 | 60 | = 4·0 | 10 | = 280·0 |
| 8 | = 0·5 | 90 | = 5·3 | 20 | = 568·0 |
| 10 | = 0·6 | 120 | = 8·0 | Gallon | Litres |
| 12 | = 0·8 | 240 | = 16·0 | 1 | = 4·536 |

### DOMESTIC MEASURES

1 teaspoonful is just over a fluid drachm or 3·5 ml.
1 dessertspoonful is about two fluid drachms.
1 tablespoonful is about half a fluid ounce or 15 ml.
1 teacupful is about five fluid ounces.
1 tumblerful is about ten fluid ounces or about half a pint.

N.B.—These measures are only approximate and should not normally be used.

## Conversion of Metric and Imperial Measures

### WEIGHTS

| Grains | × 0·0648 | = grams. |
|---|---|---|
| Grams | × 15·432 | = grains. |
| Grams | × 0·0322 | = ℥i (apoth.). |
| Grams | × 0·0353 | = oz. (avor.). |
| Kilograms | × 2·2046 | = lbs. (avor.). |
| Drachms (ʒi) | × 3·8879 | = grams. |
| Ounce (℥i) | × 31·1035 | = grams. |
| Ounce (avor.) | × 28·3495 | = grams. |
| Pounds | × 0·4536 | = kilos. |

### FLUID MEASURE

| Mils (c.c.) | × 16·8941 | = minims. |
|---|---|---|
| Mils (c.c.) | × 0·2816 | = fl. drachms. |
| Mils (c.c.) | × 0·0352 | = fl. oz. |
| Litres | × 35·1960 | = fl. oz. |
| Litres | × 1·7598 | = pints. |
| Litres | × 0·2199 | = gallons. |
| Minims | × 0·0592 | = Mils (c.c.). |
| Fl. drachms | × 3·5515 | = Mils (c.c.). |
| Fl. oz. | × 28·4123 | = Mils (c.c.). |
| Fl. oz. | × 0·0284 | = Litres. |
| Pints | × 0·5682 | = Litres. |
| Gallons | × 4·5459 | = Litres. |

### U.S.A. Liquid Measure

The minim, fluid drachm and fluid ounce of the British (Imperial) measure are slightly smaller than the corresponding measures in the U.S. Apothecaries Measure, but 16 ounces = 1 pint in U.S. measure instead of 20 ounces = 1 pint in Imperial, and therefore the British (Imperial) pint, quart and gallon are considerably larger than the corresponding U.S. measures.

To convert U.S. minims, fluid drachms or fluid ounces in British (Imperial) measure, multiply by 1·0406. To convert the British measure into U.S. measure, multiply by 0·9609.

To convert U.S. pints, quarts or gallons into British (Imperial) measure, multiply by 0·8325. To convert the British measure into U.S. measure, multiply by 1·2011.

# ALTERNATIVE NAMES OF SOME COMMON DRUGS

| Unofficial or Trade name | B.P. or Official name |
|---|---|
| Achromycin | Tetracycline |
| Albucid | Sulphacetamide |
| Amytal | Amylobarbitone |
| Anacardone | Nikethamide |
| Anthisan | Mepyramine |
| Antipar | Piperazine |
| Antistin | Antazoline |
| Apresoline | Hydrallazine |
| Argyrol | Silver protein (mild) |
| Artane | Benzhexol |
| Aureomycin | Chlortetracycline |
| Avomine | Promethazine chlorotheophyllinate |
| | |
| Benadryl | Diphenhydramine |
| Benemid | Probenecid |
| Benerva | Aneurin |
| Benzedrine | Amphetamine |
| Butazolidine | Phenylbutazone |
| | |
| Cardiazol | Leptazol |
| Cardophyllin | Aminophylline |
| Cetavlon | Cetrimide |
| Chloromycetin | Chloramphenicol |
| Choledyl | Oxtriphylline (choline theophyllinate) |
| Coramine | Nikethamide |
| Cytamen | Cyanocobalamin (Vit. $B_{12}$) |
| | |
| Dexedrine | Dextramphetamine |
| Diamox | Acetazolamide |
| Dindevan | Phenindione |
| Disprin | Soluble acetylsalicylic acid |
| Distaquaine | Procaine benzyl penicillin |
| Doriden | Glutethimide |
| Dramamine | Dimenhydrinate |
| Dromoran | Levorphanol |
| Dulcolax | Bisacodyl |
| | |
| Empirin | Acetylsalicylic acid |
| Epanutin | Phenytoin |
| Equanil | Meprobamate |
| Eserine | Physostigmine |

| Unofficial or Trade name | B.P. or Official name |
|---|---|
| Eumydrin | Atropine methonitrate |
| Evipan | Hexobarbitone |
| | |
| Femergin | Ergotamine tartrate |
| Fersolate | Ferrous sulphate |
| Flaxedil | Gallamine |
| Furadantin | Nitrofurantoin |
| | |
| Gantrisin | Sulphafurazole |
| Gardenal | Phenobarbitone |
| | |
| Hibitane | Chlorhexidine |
| | |
| I.N.A.H. | Isoniazid |
| | |
| Lanoxin | Digoxin |
| Largactil | Chlorpromazine |
| Lethidrone | Nalorphine |
| Lipiodol | Iodized oil |
| Luminal | Phenobarbitone |
| | |
| Marzine | Cyclizine |
| Mecholyl | Methacholine |
| Medinal | Barbitone sodium |
| Megimide | Bemegride |
| Mesontoin | Methoin |
| Methedrine | Methylamphetamine |
| Miltown | Meprobamate |
| Moryl | Carbachol |
| Myanesin | Mephenesin |
| Myleran | Busulphan |
| Myocrisin | Aurothiomalate |
| Mysoline | Primidone |
| | |
| Nembutal | Pentobarbitone |
| Neo-epinine | Isoprenaline |
| Neo-mercazole | Carbimazole |
| Novocain | Procaine |
| | |
| Oblivon | Methyl pentynol |
| Ostelin | Calciferol |
| | |
| Paludrine | Proguanil |
| Pentothal | Thiopentone sodium |
| Phanodorm | Cyclobarbitone |
| Phenergan | Promethazine |

| Unofficial or Trade name | B.P. or Official name |
|---|---|
| Physeptone | Methadone, (Amidone) |
| Pipanol | Benzhexol |
| Pitocin | Oxytocin |
| Pituitrin | Posterior pituinary |
| Pronestyl | Procainamide |
| Prostigmin | Neostigmine |
| Priscol | Tolazoline |
| Prominal | Methyl phenobarbitone |
| Protargol | Silver protein |
| Pycazide | Isoniazid |
| | |
| Redoxon | Ascorbic acid |
| Rimifon | Isoniazid |
| | |
| Salyrgan | Mersalyl |
| Seconal | Quinalbarbitone |
| Serpasil | Reserpine |
| Soneryl | Butobarbitone |
| Stovarsol | Acetarsol |
| Sulfasuxidine | Succinyl sulphathiazole |
| Sulfathalidine | Phthalyl sulphathiazole |
| Sulphamezathine | Sulphadimidine |
| Sulphatriad | Trisulphonamide |
| | |
| Terramycin | Oxytetracycline |
| Tetracyn | Tetracycline |
| Thephorin | Phenindamine |
| Tridione | Troxidone |
| Trilene | Trichlorethyline |
| | |
| Urolucosil | Sulphamethiazole |
| | |
| Welldorm | Dichloralphenazone |
| | |
| Xylocaine | Lignocaine |

N.B.—Fuller lists are given in The British National Formulary and unofficial publications such as Mims.

# TABLE OF ADULT DOSES

(See also Text)

N.B.  I.V.=Intravenous.    I.M.=Intramuscular.
Subcut.=Subcutaneous or hypodermic.

| | IMPERIAL | METRIC up to |
|---|---|---|
| Acetazolamide ('Diamox') . . . | gr. 2 to 4 | 500 mg. |
| Acetomenaphthone (Vitamin K) . | gr. $\frac{1}{6}$ to 1 | 60 mg. |
| Acetylcholine Chloride . . . | gr. $1\frac{1}{2}$ (approx.) | 0·1 gram. |

## ACIDS

| | | |
|---|---|---|
| Acetic (dilute) . . . . . | dr. $\frac{1}{2}$ to 1 | 4 ml. |
| Acetylsalicylic (Aspirin) . . | gr. 5 to 15 | 1 gram |
| Ascorbic (Vitamin C) . . . | gr. $1\frac{1}{2}$ to 4 | 0·25 gram |
| Folic . . . . . . | gr. $\frac{1}{6}$ to $\frac{1}{3}$ | 20 mg. |
| Hydrochloric (dilute) . . . | m. 5 to 60 | 4 ml. |
| Mandelic . . . . . . | gr. 30 to 60 | 4 grams |
| Niconitinic . . . . . | gr. $\frac{3}{4}$ to $1\frac{1}{2}$ | 0·1 gram |
| Salicylic . . . . . . | gr. 5 to 10 | 0·6 gram |
| Tartaric . . . . . . | gr. 5 to 30 | 2 grams |

| | | |
|---|---|---|
| Amylobarbitone (Amytal) . . | gr. $1\frac{1}{2}$ to 5 | 0·3 gram |
| Amylobarbitone Sodium (Sod. Amytal) | gr. 3 to 10 | 0·6 gram |
| ,, ,, (*Intravenous*) . | gr. 5 to 15 | 1 gram |
| Aloxidone ('Malidone') *daily* . . | gr. 5 to 10 | 600 mg. |
| Aminometridine ('Mictine'), *daily* . | 200 to 800 mg. | |
| Aminophylline (*I.M. I.V.*) . . | gr. $1\frac{1}{2}$ to 8 | 10 mg. |
| Ammonium Bromide . . . . | gr. 5 to 30 | 2 grams |
| ,, Carbonate . . . | gr. 5 to 10 | 0·6 gram |
| ,, Chloride , . . | gr. 5 to 60 | 4 grams |
| Amphetamine Sulph. (Benzedrine) . | gr. $\frac{1}{12}$ to $\frac{1}{6}$ | 10 mg. |
| ,, ,, (*Injection*) . | gr. $\frac{1}{24}$ to $\frac{1}{6}$ | 10 mg. |
| Amyl Nitrite (*Inhalation*) . . . | m. 2 to 5 | 0·3 ml. |
| Adrenocorticotrophic Hormone (ACTH) (*I.M.*) | gr. $\frac{5}{12}$ to $\frac{2}{3}$ | 100 mg. |
| Aneurine Hydrochloride (Vitamin B₁) . | gr. $\frac{1}{30}$ to $\frac{3}{4}$ | 50 mg. |
| Antazoline ('Antistin') . . . | gr. $1\frac{1}{2}$ to 3 | 200 mg. |
| Antipyrine (Phenazone) . . . | gr. 5 to 10 | 0·6 gram |
| Apomorphine Hydrochloride . . | gr. $\frac{1}{12}$ to $\frac{1}{8}$ | 8 mg. |

## WATERS

| | | |
|---|---|---|
| Aqua Anethi (Aniseed) . . . | | |
| ,, Camphoræ (Camphor) . . | | |
| ,, Chloroformi (Chloroform) . | fl. oz. $\frac{1}{2}$ to 1 | 30 ml. |
| ,, Cinnamomi (Cinnamon) . . | | |
| ,, Menthæ Piperitæ (Peppermint) . | | |
| Aspirin . . . . . . | gr. 5 to 15 | 1 gram |
| Atropine: Atropine Sulphate . . | gr. $\frac{1}{240}$ to $\frac{1}{60}$ | 1 mg. |
| Atropine Methonitrate (Eumydrin) . | gr. $\frac{1}{60}$ to $\frac{1}{30}$ | 2 mg. |
| Barbitone Sodium (Medinal) . . | gr. 5 to 10 | 0·6 gram |
| Barbitone (Veronal) . . . | gr. 5 to 10 | 0·6 gram |

|  | IMPERIAL | METRIC up to |
|---|---|---|
| Benzhexol . . . . (daily) | increased from 2 mg. up to 15 mg |  |
| Benzocaine (Anæsthesin) . . . | gr. 5 to 10 | 0·6 gram |
| Bismuth Carbonate . . . | gr. 10 to 30 | 2 grams |
| Bismuth Oxychloride . . . | gr. 10 to 30 | 2 grams |
| ,, ,, (intramuscular) | gr. $1\frac{1}{2}$ to 3 | 0·2 gram |
| ,, precipitated (intramuscular) | gr. $1\frac{1}{2}$ to 3 | 0·2 gram |
| ,, Salicylate . . . . | gr. 10 to 30 | 2 grams |
| ,, Subnitrate . . . . | gr. 5 to 20 | 1·2 gram |
| Butobarbitone ('Soneryl') . . | gr. 1 to 2 | 120 mg. |
| Caffeine . . . . . | gr. 2 to 5 | 0·3 gram |
| ,, Citrate . . . . | gr. 2 to 10 | 0·6 gram |
| Calciferol (Vitamin D) . | gr. $\frac{1}{2400}$ to $\frac{1}{800}$ | 0·075 mg. |
| Calcium Carbonate . . . . | gr. 15 to 60 | 4 grams |
| ,, Chloride . . . . | gr. 10 to 30 | 2 grams |
| ,, ,, (intramuscular) . | gr. $\frac{1}{2}$ to $1\frac{1}{2}$ | 0·1 gram |
| ,, ,, (intravenous) . | gr. 5 to 15 | 1 gram |
| ,, Gluconate . . . | gr. 30 to 60 | 4 grams |
| ,, Hydroxide . . . | gr. 5 to 15 | 1 gram |
| ,, Lactate . . . | gr. 15 to 60 | 4 grams |
| Calomel . . . . . | gr. $\frac{1}{2}$ to 3 | 0·2 gram |
| Carbachol (Moryl) . . . | gr. $\frac{1}{64}$ to $\frac{1}{16}$ | 4 mg. |
| ,, ,, (subcutaneous) . | gr. $\frac{1}{240}$ to $\frac{1}{120}$ | 0·5 mg. |
| Carbimazole (therapeutic daily) . | 20-40 mg. |  |
| ,, (maintenance daily) . | 5-15 mg. |  |
| Carbon Tetrachloride . . . | m. 30 to 60 | 4 ml. |
| Chloralformamide (Chloralamide) | gr. 15 to 45 | 3 grams |
| Chloral Hydrate . . . | gr. 5 to 30 | 2 grams |
| Chlorbutol (Chloretone) . . | gr. 5 to 20 | 1·2 gram |
| Chlorpromazine (oral daily) . . | up to 150 mg. |  |
| ,, (intramuscular) . . |  | 50 mg. |
| Cocaine Hydrochloride . . . | gr. $\frac{1}{8}$ to $\frac{1}{4}$ | 16 mg. |
| Codeine: Codeine Phosphate . . | gr. $\frac{1}{6}$ to 1 | 60 mg. |
| Colchicine . . . . | gr. $\frac{1}{120}$ to $\frac{1}{60}$ | 1 mg. |
| Confection of Senna . . | gr. 60 to 120 | 8 grams |
| Copper sulphate (emetic) . . | gr. 5 to 10 | 0·6 gram |
| Cortisone Acetate Oral or I.M.) . | gr. 1 to 5 | 300 mg. |
| Creosote . . . . . | m. 2 to 10 | 0·6 ml. |
| Creta (Chalk) . . . . | gr. 15 to 60 | 4 grams |
| Cyclizine ('Marzine') . . . | gr. $\frac{2}{5}$ to $\frac{3}{4}$ | 50 mg. |
| Deoxycortone Acetate (I.M.) . . | gr. $\frac{1}{30}$ to $\frac{1}{6}$ | 10 mg. |
| Diamorphine Hydrochloride (Heroin) . | gr. $\frac{1}{24}$ to 0 | 8 mg. |
| Digitalin (amorphous) (German) . | gr. $\frac{1}{2}$ to 1 | 60 mg. |
| ,, (crystalline) (French) . | gr. $\frac{1}{600}$ to $\frac{1}{60}$ | 1 mg. |
| Digitalis (powdered) or Folia (leaves) . | gr. $\frac{1}{2}$ to $1\frac{1}{2}$ | 0·1 gram |
| ,, ,, (single dose) . | gr. 3 to 10 | 0·6 gram |
| Digoxin (oral, initial dose) . . | gr. $\frac{1}{60}$ to $\frac{1}{40}$ | 1·5 gram. |
| ,, (oral, maintenance) . . | gr. $\frac{1}{240}$ | 0·25 mg. |
| ,, (intravenously) . . | gr. $\frac{1}{120}$ to $\frac{1}{60}$ | 1 mg. |
| Dimenhydrinate ('Dramamine') . | gr. $\frac{2}{5}$ to $\frac{3}{4}$ | 50 mg. |
| Diphenhydramine ('Benadryl') . | gr. $\frac{3}{4}$ to $1\frac{1}{2}$ | 100 mg. |
| Elixir Cascaræ Sagradæ . . . | m. 30 to 60 | 4 ml. |

K

| | IMPERIAL | METRIC up to |
|---|---|---|
| Emetine et Bismuth Iodide . . . | gr. 1 to 3 | 0·2 gram |
| „ Hydrochloride (*emetic*) . | gr. $\frac{1}{12}$ to $\frac{1}{6}$ | 10 mg. |
| „ „ (*Subcut. or I.M.*) | gr. $\frac{1}{2}$ to 1 | 60 mg. |
| Emulsion, Cod Liver Oil . . . | m. 30 to 180 | 12 ml. |
| „ Vitamin Oil . . . | m. 30 to 180 | 12 ml. |
| Ephedrine Hydrochloride . . . | gr. $\frac{1}{4}$ to $1\frac{1}{2}$ | 0·1 gram |
| Ergometrine (*intramuscular*) . . | gr. $\frac{1}{240}$ to $\frac{1}{60}$ | 1 mg. |
| Ergometrine (*intravenous*) . . | gr. $\frac{1}{480}$ to $\frac{1}{240}$ | 0·5 mg. |
| Ergotamine Tartrate (*Subcut. or I.M.*) . | gr. $\frac{1}{240}$ to $\frac{1}{120}$ | 0·5 mg. |
| Ergot (prepared) . . . . | gr. $2\frac{1}{2}$ to 8 | 0·5 gram |
| Ergotoxine . . . . . | gr. $\frac{1}{100}$ to $\frac{1}{60}$ | 1·2 mg. |
| Erythrol Tetranitrate . . . | gr. $\frac{1}{4}$ to 1 | 60 mg. |
| Ethinyloestradiol (*daily*) . . . | —— | 0·02 to 0·1 mg. |
| Eserine (*see* Physostigmine) | | |
| Ferri et Ammonii Citras . . . | gr. 5 to 30 | 2 grams |
| „ Sulphas . . . . | gr. 1 to 5 | 0·3 gram |
| Glycerin . . . . . | dr. 1 to 2 | 8 ml. |
| Glyceryl Trinitrate (*Sublingual*) . | gr. $\frac{1}{120}$ | 0·5 mg. |
| Guaiacol Carbonate . . . | gr. 5 to 15 | 1 gram |
| Heparin (*I.V.*) . . . . | 6000 to 12,000 units | |
| Hexamethonium Bromide . . | gr. 4 to 8 | 0·5 gram |
| „ „ (*Subcut. or I.M.*) | gr. $\frac{2}{3}$ to $\frac{3}{4}$ | 50 mg. |
| Hexamine . . . . . | gr. 10 to 30 | 2 grams |
| Histamine Acid Phosphate . . | gr. $\frac{1}{120}$ to $\frac{1}{60}$ | 1 mg. |
| Homatropine Hydrobromide . . | gr. $\frac{1}{64}$ to $\frac{1}{32}$ | 2 mg. |
| Hydrargyri Perchloridum (Corrosive sublimate) . . . . | gr. $\frac{1}{32}$ to $\frac{1}{16}$ | 4 mg. |
| Hydrargyri Subchloridum (Calomel) . | gr. $\frac{1}{2}$ to 3 | 0·2 gram |
| Hydrargyrum cum Creta (Grey powder) | gr. 1 to 5 | 0·3 gram |
| Hyoscine Hydrobromide . . | gr. $\frac{1}{200}$ to $\frac{1}{100}$ | 0·6 mg. |
| Indicarmine (*subcutaneous*) . . | gr. $\frac{3}{4}$ to $1\frac{1}{2}$ | 0·1 gram |
| „ (*intravenous*) . . | gr. $\frac{1}{8}$ to $\frac{1}{4}$ | 16 mg. |
| Infusions (various) average dose . | fl. oz. $\frac{1}{2}$ to 1 | 30 ml. |

### INJECTIONS, B.P.

| | IMPERIAL | METRIC up to |
|---|---|---|
| Injectio Adrenalini (1 in 1000) . | m. 2 to 8 | 0·5 ml. |
| „ Bismuthi . . . | m. 8 to 15 | 1 ml. |
| „ Calcii Gluconatis . . | m. 150 to 300 | 20 ml. |
| „ Leptazoli (Cardiazol) . | m. 8 to 15 | 1 ml. |
| „ Mersalyli . . . | m. 8 to 30 | 2 ml. |
| „ Nikethamidi (Coramine) . | m. 15 to 60 | 4 ml. |
| „ Quininæ et Urethani . | m. 8 to 75 | 5 ml. |
| „ Sodii Morrhuatis . . | m. 8 to 75 | 5 ml. |
| Insulin . . . . . | 5 to 100 units | |
| Iodophthalein (Gall bladder dye) . | up to 75 grains | |
| Ipecacuanha (powdered) (*expectorant*) . | gr. $\frac{1}{2}$ to 2 | 0·12 gram |
| „ „ (*emetic*) . | gr. 15 to 30 | 2 grams |
| Isoniazid (*daily*) . . . | —— | 150 to 400 mg. |
| Isoprenaline (*sublingual*) . . | gr. $\frac{1}{8}$ to $\frac{1}{2}$ | 30 mg. |
| Kaolin (light) . . . . | oz. $\frac{1}{2}$ to 2 | 60 grams |
| Leptazol (Cardiazol) . . . | gr. $\frac{3}{4}$ to $1\frac{1}{2}$ | 0·1 gram |

| | Imperial | Metric up to |
|---|---|---|
| **Liquores** (Solutions) | | |
| Liquor Ammonia Acetatis Dil. . . . | dr. 2 to 8 | 30 ml. |
| ,, ,, ,, Fort. . . . | m. 15 to 60 | 4 ml. |
| ,, Arsenicalis . . . . . . . | m. 2 to 8 | 0·5 ml. |
| ,, Calciferolis (1000 to 3000 units) | m. 5 to 15 | 1 ml. |
| ,, Calcii Hydroxidi . . . . | fl. oz. 1 to 4 | 120 ml. |
| ,, Ferri Perchloridi . . . . . | m. 5 to 15 | 1 ml. |
| ,, Glycerylis Trinitratis . . . . | m. $\frac{1}{2}$ to 2 | 0·12 ml. |
| ,, Hydrarg. Perchlor. . . . . | m. 30 to 60 | 4 ml. |
| ,, Iodi Aquosus (Lugol's iodine) . | m. 5 to 15 | 1 ml. |
| ,, ,, Mitis . . . . . . . | m. 5 to 30 | 2 ml. |
| ,, Magnesii Bicarbonaris . . . | fl. oz. 1 to 2 | 60 ml. |
| ,, Morphinæ Hydrochlor. . . . | m. 5 to 30 | 2 ml. |
| ,, Potassii Hydroxidi . . . . | m. 10 to 30 | 2 ml. |
| ,, Quininæ Ammoniatis . . . . | m. 30 to 60 | 4 ml. |
| ,, Strychninæ Hydrochl. . . . | m. 3 to 12 | 0·8 ml. |
| ,, Vitamini A Conc. (2500-12,500 units) . . . . . . . | m. 1 to 5 | 0·3 ml. |
| ,, Vitamini D Conc. (250-1500 units) | m. $\frac{1}{2}$ to 3 | 0·2 ml. |
| ,, Vitamin A et D Conc. (A=2500-12,500 units, D=250-1250 unit) | m. 1 to 5 | 0·3 ml. |
| Magnesium Carbonate (light, heavy) . | gr. 10 to 60 | 4 grams |
| ,, Oxide (light) / ,, ,, (heavy) . . | gr. 10 to 60 | 4 grams |
| ,, Sulphate . . . . . | gr. 30 to 240 | 16 grams |
| ,, Trisilicate . . . . . | gr. 5 to 30 | 2 grams |
| Mepacrine Hydrochloride ('Atebrin') . | gr. $\frac{3}{4}$ to $1\frac{1}{2}$ | 0·1 gram |
| Meprobamate . . . . . . . . | gr. 6 | 400 mg. |
| Mepyramine maleate ('Anthisan'), daily | 300-800 mg. | |
| Methadone Hydrochloride ('Physeptone') | gr. $\frac{1}{12}$ to $\frac{1}{6}$ | 10 mg. |
| Methylamphetamine ('Methedrine') . | gr. $\frac{1}{24}$ to $\frac{1}{6}$ | 10 mg. |
| ,, (*I.M. or I.V.*) . | gr. $\frac{1}{6}$ to $\frac{1}{2}$ | 10 mg. |
| Methylsulphonal . . . . . . . | gr. 5 to 20 | 1·2 gram |
| Methyltestosterone (daily) . . . . | —— | 50 mg. |
| Methylthiouracil . . . . . . . | gr. $\frac{3}{4}$ to 3 | 0·2 gram |
| Mist. Magnesii Hydroxidi . . . | dr. 1 to 4 | 16 ml. |
| ,, Sennæ Co. . . . . . . . | fl. oz. 1 to 2 | 60 ml. |
| Morphine Hydrochloride . . . . | gr. $\frac{1}{8}$ to $\frac{1}{3}$ | 0·02 gram |
| ,, Sulphate . . . . . . | gr. $\frac{1}{8}$ to $\frac{1}{3}$ | 0·02 gram |
| Mucilage of Acacia . . . . . | dr. 1 to 4 | 16 ml. |
| ,, Tragacanth . . . . . | dr. 1 to 4 | 16 ml. |
| Nalorphine Hydrochloride (*I.V.*) . . | gr. $\frac{1}{6}$ to $\frac{3}{5}$ | 40 mg. |
| Neoarsphenamine (*intravenously*) . . | gr. $2\frac{1}{2}$ to 14 | 1 gram |
| Neostigmine (*Subcut. or I.M.*) . . . | gr. $\frac{1}{120}$ to $\frac{1}{30}$ | 2 mg. |
| Nicotinamide . . . . . . . | gr. $\frac{1}{3}$ to $1\frac{1}{2}$ | 0·1 gram |
| Nikethamide (Coramine) . . . . | gr. 3 to 8 | 0·5 gram |
| ,, (*intravenously*) . . . | gr. 8 to 20 | 1·25 gram |
| Nitrofurantoin ('Furadantin') . . . | 50-150 mg. | |
| **Oils** | | |
| Oleum Anethi (Dill) . . . . . | m. 1 to 3 | 0·2 ml. |
| ,, Anisi (Aniseed) . . . . . | m. 1 to 3 | 0·2 ml. |

| | IMPERIAL | METRIC up to |
|---|---|---|
| Oleum Arachis | fl. oz. $\frac{1}{2}$ to 1 | 30 ml. |
| ,, Cajuputi | m. 1 to 3 | 0·2 ml. |
| ,, Caryophylli (Clove) | m. 1 to 3 | 0·2 ml. |
| ,, Chenopodii | m. 3 to 15 | 1 ml. |
| ,, Eucalypti | m. 1 to 3 | 0·2 ml. |
| ,, Hippoglossi (Halibut) (A=1500-7500 *units*, D=3000 *units approx.*) | m. 1 to 5 | 0·3 ml. |
| ,, Menthæ Pip (Peppermint) | m. 1 to 3 | 0·2 ml. |
| ,, Morrhuæ (Cod Liver) | m. 30 to 120 | 8 ml. |
| ,, Olivæ | fl. oz. $\frac{1}{2}$ to 1 | 30 ml. |
| ,, Ricini (Castor Oil) | dr. 1 to 4 | 16 ml. |
| ,, Terebinthinæ (Turpentine) | m. 3 to 10 | 0·6 ml. |
| ,, ,, (*Anthelmintic*) | m. 120 to 240 | 16 ml. |
| ,, Vitaminatum (*Prophylactic*, A = 1000-2000 *units*, D=100-200 *units*) | m. 15 to 30 | 2 ml. |
| (*Therapeutic*, A = 3000-6000 *units*, D=300-600 *units*) | m. 45 to 90 | 6 ml. |
| Œstradiol Benzoate (1000-50,000 units) | gr. $\frac{1}{600}$ to $\frac{1}{12}$ | 5 mg. |
| Œstrone (1000-100,000 units) | gr. $\frac{1}{600}$ to $\frac{1}{6}$ | 10 mg. |
| Pamaquin | gr. $\frac{1}{6}$ to $\frac{1}{2}$ | 20 mg. |
| Paraffin (Liquid) | fl. oz. $\frac{1}{4}$ to 1 | 30 ml. |
| Paraldehyde | dr. $\frac{1}{2}$ to 2 | 8 ml. |
| Pentobarbitone Soluble (Nembutal) | gr. $1\frac{1}{2}$ to 3 | 0·2 gram |
| Pepsin | gr. 5 to 10 | 0·6 gram |
| Pethidine Hydrochloride | gr. $\frac{1}{2}$ to $1\frac{1}{2}$ | 0·1 gram |
| Phemitone (Prominal) | gr. $\frac{1}{2}$ to 6 | 0·4 gram |
| Phenacetin | gr. 5 to 10 | 0·6 gram |
| Phenazone | gr. 5 to 10 | 0·6 gram |
| Phenobarbitone (Luminal) | gr. $\frac{1}{2}$ to 2 | 0·12 gram |
| ,, Sodium (*I.M. or I.V.*) | gr. 1 to 3 | 0·2 gram |
| Phenolphthalein | gr. 1 to 5 | 0·3 gram |
| Phenylbutazone ('Butazolidine') *daily* | 200-400 mg. | |
| Phenytoin Sodium (Epanutin) | gr. $\frac{3}{4}$ to $1\frac{1}{2}$ | 100 mg. |
| Pholedrine Sulphate | gr. $\frac{1}{6}$ to $\frac{1}{3}$ | 20 mg. |
| Physeptone (Amidone) | gr. $\frac{1}{12}$ to $\frac{1}{6}$ | 10 mg. |
| Physostigmine Sulphate | gr. $\frac{1}{100}$ to $\frac{1}{50}$ | 1·2 mg. |
| Picrotoxin (*I.M. or I.V.*) | gr. $\frac{1}{100}$ to $\frac{1}{10}$ | 6 mg. |
| Pilocarpine Nitrate | gr. $\frac{1}{20}$ to $\frac{1}{2}$ | 12 mg. |

PILLS

| | IMPERIAL | METRIC |
|---|---|---|
| Potassium Bicarbonate | gr. 15 to 30 | 2 grams |
| ,, Bromide | gr. 5 to 30 | 2 grams |
| ,, Chlorate | gr. 5 to 10 | 0·6 gram |
| ,, Citrate | gr. 15 to 60 | 4 grams |
| ,, Iodide | gr. 5 to 30 | 2 grams |
| ,, Permanganate | gr. 1 to 3 | 0·2 gram |
| ,, Sulphate | gr. 15 to 45 | 3 grams |
| Procaine Hydrochloride | gr. $\frac{1}{2}$ to 2 | 0·12 gram |
| ,, ,, (*subcutaneously*) | up to gr. 15 | 1 gram |
| ,, ,, (*intrathecally*) | up to gr. $2\frac{1}{2}$ | 0·15 gram |
| Progesterone (1-5 units) | gr. $\frac{1}{60}$ to $\frac{1}{12}$ | 5 mg. |

|  | IMPERIAL | METRIC up to |
|---|---|---|
| Proguanil (Paludrine) daily . . . | gr. $1\frac{1}{2}$ to 6 | 0·4 gram |
| Propantheline ('Probanthine') . . | 15-30 mg. | |

### POWDERS

|  | IMPERIAL | METRIC |
|---|---|---|
| Pulvis Cretæ Aromaticus . . . | gr. 10 to 60 | 4 grams |
| „ „ Aromaticus c̄ Opio . . | gr. 10 to 60 | 4 grams |
| „ Glycyrrh. Comp. . . . . | gr. 60 to 120 | 8 grams |
| „ Ipecacuanhæ et Opii (Dover's) . | gr. 5 to 10 | 0·6 gram |
| „ Rhei Comp. . . . . . | gr. 10 to 60 | 4 grams |
| Riboflavine . . . . . . | gr. $\frac{1}{60}$ to $\frac{1}{6}$ | 10 mg. |
| Quinalbarbitone Sodium (Seconal Sod.) | gr. $\frac{3}{4}$ to 3 | 0·2 gram |
| Quinidine Sulphate . . . . . | gr. 1 to 5 | 0·3 gram |
| Quinine Bisulphate . . . . . | gr. 1 to 10 | 0·6 gram |
| „ Dihydrochloride . . . | gr. 1 to 10 | 0·6 gram |
| (*intravenously* or *intramuscularly*) . . . . . | gr. 5 to 10 | 0·6 gram |
| „ Sulphate . . . . | gr. 1 to 10 | 0·6 gram |
| Saccharin Soluble . . . . . | gr. $\frac{1}{2}$ to 2 | 0·12 gram |
| Santonin . . . . . . . | gr. 1 to 3 | 0·2 gram |
| Scopolamine (*see* Hyoscine) . . . | | |
| Senna Leaves . . . . . . | gr. 10 to 30 | 2 grams |
| Sodium Bicarbonate . . . . | gr. 15 to 60 | 4 grams |
| „ Bromide . . . . . | gr. 5 to 30 | 2 grams |
| „ Citrate . . . . . | gr. 15 to 60 | 4 grams |
| „ Iodide . . . . . | gr. 5 to 30 | 2 grams |
| „ Nitrite . . . . . | gr. $\frac{1}{2}$ to 2 | 0·12 gram |
| „ Phosphate . . . | gr. 30 to 240 | 16 grams |
| „ „ (Acid) . . | gr. 30 to 60 | 4 grams |
| „ Phosphate . . . | gr. 30 to 240 | 16 grams |
| „ „ (Acid) . . | gr. 30 to 60 | 4 grams |
| „ „ (Effervescent) . | gr. 60 to 240 | 16 grams |
| „ Salicylate . . . . | gr. 10 to 30 | 2 grams |
| „ Sulphate . . . . | gr. 30 to 240 | 16 grams |
| „ „ (Effervescent) . | gr. 60 to 240 | 16 grams |
| „ „ (Dry) . . . | gr. 15 to 120 | 8 grams |
| „ Thiosulphate (*subcutaneously, intramuscularly* or *intravenously*) . | gr. 5 to 15 | 1·0 gram |
| Spiritus Ammon. Arom. . . . . | m. 15 to 60 | 4 ml. |
| Stibophen (Fouadin) (*I.V.*) . . | gr. $1\frac{1}{2}$ to 5 | 0·3 gram |
| Stilbœstrol . . . . . . | gr. $\frac{1}{120}$ to $\frac{1}{30}$ | 2 mg. |
| Strophanthin (*I.M.* or *I.V.*) . . | gr. $\frac{1}{240}$ to $\frac{1}{60}$ | 1 mg. |
| Strophanthin G (Ouabain) . . | gr. $\frac{1}{600}$ to $\frac{1}{120}$ | 0·5 mg. |
| Strychnine Hydrochloride . . | gr. $\frac{1}{32}$ to $\frac{1}{8}$ | 8 mg. |
| Sulphadiazine . . . . . | gr. 8 to 30 | 2 grams |
| Sulphapyridine . . . . . | gr. 8 to 30 | 2 grams |
| Sulphathiazole . . . . . | gr. 8 to 30 | 2 grams |
| Sulphaguanidine . . . . . | gr. 8 to 30 | 2 grams |
| Sulpharsphenamine (*subcutaneously intramuscularly*) . . . . | gr. $1\frac{1}{2}$ to 10 | 0·6 gram |

|  | | IMPERIAL | METRIC up to |
|---|---|---|---|
| **SYRUPS** | | | |
| Syrupus Aurantii (Orange) . . . | | dr. ½ to 2 | 8 ml. |
|     ,,    Codeinæ Phosphatis . . . | | dr. ½ to 2 | 8 ml. |
|     ,,    Ferri Phosphatis Co. . . | | dr. ½ to 2 | 8 ml. |
|     ,,    ,,  Phosp. c̄ . . . | | dr. ½ to 1 | 4 ml. |
|     ,,    Quin. et Strych. (Easton) | | | |
|     ,,    Scillæ . . . . . | | dr. ½ to 1 | 4 ml. |
|     ,,    Sennæ . . . . . . | | dr. ½ to 2 | 8 ml. |
|     ,,    Tolutanus . . . . . | | dr. ½ to 2 | 8 ml. |
| Thyroid . . . . . . | | gr. ½ to 2 | 1·2 gram |
| Tolazoline ('Priscol') . . . | | gr. ⅛ to ¼ | 50 mg. |
| Troxidone ('Tridione') . . . | | gr. 1½ to 6 | 0·4 gram |
| Tryparsamide (*subcutaneously, intramuscularly or intravenously*) . . . | | gr. 15 to 30 | 2 grams |
| Urea . . . . . . . | | gr. 15 to 240 | 16 grams |
| Urethane . . . . . . | | gr. 15 to 30 | 2 grams |
| Zinc Oxide . . . . . | | gr. 5 to 10 | 0·6 gram |
|   ,,  Sulphate . . . . | | gr. 1 to 3 | 0·2 gram |
|   ,,    ,,  (*emetic*) . . . | | gr. 10 to 30 | 2 grams |

# INDEX

Acetarsol, 214
Acetylcholine, 176
Achromycin, 236
Acid, acetic, 38
   acetyl salicylic, 153
   ascorbic, 183
   boric, 38
   carbolic, 41
   chromic, 53
   hydrochloric, 37, 53, 67
   folic, 183
   mandelic, 131
   nicotinic, 183
   nitric, 37, 53
   salicylic, 38
   tannic, 37
Acids and alkalis, 37
Acriflavine, 48
Addison's disease, 197
Adrenaline, 119, 173
A.C.T.H., 201
Aerosporin, 237
Agar, 72
Agranulocytosis, 103, 194, 228
Alcohol, 220
Alcohols, 40
Alcopar, 83
Aleudrin, 119
Alkaloids, 3
Aloes, 74
Aludrox, 67
Aluminium hydroxide, 67
Amethocaine, 165
Amidopyrine, 155
Aminophylline, 120
Amphetamine, 163
Amyl nitrite, 94
Anacardone, 93
Anadin, 154
Anæsthesin, 123
Anæsthetics, general, 136
   local, 163
   spinal, 166

Anahæmin, 101
Anaphylactic shock, 251
Androgens, 206
Aneurine, 181
Anhydrotics, 60
Antacids, 66
Anthelmintics, 81
Anthisan, 97
Antihistamines, 97
Anthrax (serum), 254
Antibiotics, 4, 229
Anti-coagulants, 109
Antiparasitics, 52, 79
Antiphlogistine, 57
Antipyretics, 60
Antiseptics, 33, 52
   (pulmonary), 120
   (urinary), 130
Anti-snake venom serum, 255
Antispasmodics, 119
Antistin, 97
Aperients, 69
Applications, 11
Apomorphine, 64
Aquæ, 11
Arsenic, 213
Aspirin, 153
Asterol, 53
Astringents, 56
Atebrin, 217
Atropine, 177, 210
A.T. 10, 195
Aureomycin, 235
Auristillæ, 11
Avertin, 144
Avomine, 66
Axerophthol, 180

Bacillus coli infections, 130
Bacitracin, 237
B.A.L., 220
Barbiturates, 148
Barium meal, enema, 68

287